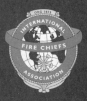

International Association of Fire Chiefs

EXAM PREP

Paramedic

D1298709

By Dr. Ben A. Hirst,
Performance Training
Systems

JONES AND BARTLETT PUBLISHERS
Sudbury, Massachusetts
BOSTON   TORONTO   LONDON   SINGAPORE

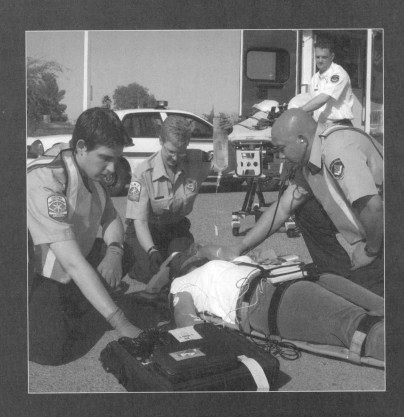

Jones and Bartlett Publishers
World Headquarters
40 Tall Pine Drive
Sudbury, MA 01776
978-443-5000
www.jbpub.com

Jones and Bartlett Publishers Canada
6339 Ormindale Way
Mississauga, Ontario L5V 1J2
Canada

Jones and Bartlett Publishers
International
Barb House, Barb Mews
London W6 7PA
United Kingdom

International Association of
Fire Chiefs
4025 Fair Ridge Drive
Fairfax, VA 22033
www.IAFC.org

Performance Training
Systems, Inc.
760 U.S. Highway One, Suite 101
North Palm Beach, FL 33408
www.FireTestBanks.com

Jones and Bartlett's books and products are available through most bookstores and online booksellers. To contact Jones and Bartlett Publishers directly, call 800-832-0034, fax 978-443-8000, or visit our website www.jbpub.com.

Substantial discounts on bulk quantities of Jones and Bartlett's publications are available to corporations, professional associations, and other qualified organizations. For details and specific discount information, contact the special sales department at Jones and Bartlett via the above contact information or send an email to specialsales@jbpub.com.

Editorial Credits
Author: Dr. Ben A. Hirst

Production Credits
Chief Executive Officer: Clayton E. Jones
Chief Operating Officer: Donald W. Jones, Jr.
President, Higher Education and Professional Publishing:
    Robert W. Holland, Jr.
V.P., Sales and Marketing: William J. Kane
V.P., Production and Design: Anne Spencer
V.P., Manufacturing and Inventory Control: Therese Connell
Publisher, Public Safety Group: Kimberly Brophy

Editorial Assistant: Amanda Brandt
Production Editor: Karen Ferreira
Director of Marketing: Alisha Weisman
Senior Photo Researcher: Kimberly Potvin
Cover Design: Kristin E. Ohlin
Interior Design: Anne Spencer
Composition: Northeast Compositors
Printing and Binding: Courier Stoughton

Copyright © 2007 by Jones and Bartlett Publishers, Inc. and Performance Training Systems, Inc.

Photo Credits
Cover photo © Jones and Bartlett Publishers. Courtesy of MIEMMS.

ISBN-13: 978-0-7637-4216-4
ISBN-10: 0-7637-4216-3
6048

The procedures in this text are based on the most current recommendations of responsible sources. The publisher and Performance Training Systems, Inc. make no guarantees as to, and assume no responsibility for the correctness, sufficiency, or completeness of such information or recommendations. Other or additional safety measures may be required under particular circumstances. This text is intended solely as a guide to the appropriate procedures to be employed when responding to an emergency. It is not intended as a statement of the procedures required in any particular situation, because circumstances can vary widely from one emergency to another. Nor is it intended that this text shall in any way advise firefighting personnel concerning legal authority to perform the activities or procedures discussed. Such local determination should be made only with the aid of legal counsel.

Printed in the United States of America
10 09 08 07 06   10 9 8 7 6 5 4 3 2 1

CONTENTS

ACKNOWLEDGMENTS

More than nine paramedics have contributed to the development, validation, revision, and updating of the test items included in this *Exam Prep* book. Their efforts are valued because of the credibility they provided. A special thanks goes to the recent Technical Review Committee for Paramedics for validating and updating the test items to the latest DOT Standard and latest publications: Chris O. Seay, Paramedic/Firefighter, Palm Beach County Fire Rescue, Florida; Lt. Todd Lynch, Paramedic/Firefighter, Delray Beach Fire Department, Florida; Lt. Walter Hirst, Paramedic/Firefighter, Delray Beach Fire Department, Florida; Edmund Beardsley, Paramedic/Firefighter, Delray Beach Fire Department, Florida; John Connolly, Paramedic/Firefighter, Delray Beach Fire Department, Florida. These individuals worked diligently to make considerable improvements in the test items.

I want to thank my family and friends who encouraged me to continue pressing forward with the work. Without their understanding and support, I would not have been able to meet the scheduled delivery date.

Last, but not least, I express my sincere thanks to my able staff: Ellen Korn Eastwood, Administrative Assistant; Paulette Kelly, Clerical Staff; Walter Hirst, Paramedic/Firefighter and Director of Operations; Lt. Todd Lynch, Paramedic/Firefighter and Regional Sales Manager; Chris Seay, Paramedic/Firefighter and Regional Sales Manager; Ed Beardsley, Paramedic/Firefighter and Regional Sales Manager. While I was away, in complete solitude, they kept the business going.

PREFACE

The Emergency Medical Service (EMS) is facing one of the most challenging periods in its history. Local, state, provincial, national, and international government organizations are under pressure to deliver ever-increasing services. The events of September 11, 2001, continued activities and threats by terrorist organizations worldwide, recent natural disasters, and the need to maximize available funds are part of the reason most EMS organizations are examining and reinventing their roles.

The challenge of reinventing the Emergency Medical Service to provide the first response efforts includes increasing professional requirements. Organizations such as the U. S. Department of Transportation, National Registry of Emergency Medical Technicians, and National Highway Traffic Safety Administration are having a dramatic influence on raising the professional qualifications of the first line of defense for emergency response. Most of the United States use training and testing materials developed and funded by these organizations as the basis for certification of Emergency Medical Service personnel.

Qualification standards have been improved. Accreditation of training and certification are at the highest levels ever in the history of the Emergency Medical Service. These improvements are reflected in a better prepared first responder, but are not without an effect on those individuals who serve. EMS providers are being required to expand their roles, acquire new knowledge, develop new and higher-level technical skills, as well as participate in requalification and in-service training programs on a regular basis.

The aftermath of September 11, along with several major natural disasters, has had a profound effect on the Emergency Medical Service. Lessons learned, new technology, and national focus on terrorism and weapons of mass destruction are placing much greater demands on emergency scene operations. EMS personnel cannot afford to be complacent and continue to perform in the same way. Obvious dangers faced by first responders under current heightened security conditions require many adjustments in what is being taught as they prepare to operate in an emergency environment. Processes and modes of operation must be carefully examined and must be continuously monitored, changed, and updated.

Our national leaders are constantly pointing to the first responders as our "first line of defense" against acts of terror and defense of life and property from extremely dangerous weapons that have never been used extensively in our history. Several major disasters such as hurricanes, tornadoes, wildland fires, flooding, major injury incidents, and earthquakes have raised the awareness of planners, first responders, and hospitals regarding their response and mediation capabilities.

Some EMS programs are steeped in tradition. One thing that must happen is to question our traditions and our thinking to bring our knowledge, skills, and abilities in line with the demands of today's real world.

Many things have been learned from the September 11 attack on America. Some of these lessons learned were the result of our reluctance to change processes and procedures, i.e., our traditions. As great as our tradition is, we in the EMS industry must not stop reflecting on the paramount reasons for our existence, which is to provide quality care, save lives, and perform our tasks with personal safety as the number one concern.

These are very important reasons to exist, to continuously improve, and to move from a good EMS to a great EMS.

A few words about knowing vital strategic and tactical information are in order. There are organizations that focus a lot of their training time and effort on the performance side of EMS. That is essential and is the bottom line for developing skilled paramedics. The dark side of this approach to training is a lack of emphasis on key knowledge requirements. Often, it is not what we did or did not do as paramedics, but what we could have done if we had a strong base of knowledge that helps to analyze and detect a need for action outside the routine tasks. How many times does Plan A go wrong at the emergency scene? How well do we transition from Plan A to Plan B or Plan C? Are our emergency incident communications adequate, timely, precise, and getting to the right people? These questions may never be answered, but they do require the Emergency Medical Service as a whole, and each responder in particular, to focus equally on the knowledge portion of emergency responses to help improve the performance side of our tasks.

Pre-planning for an emergency target hazard is important; knowing what can go wrong is essential. Knowledge is the potential power we must acquire to make important adjustments during the emergency incident, to continuously size up the situations, and to alter our plan of action as needed and required.

Our supervisors, responders, and support personnel must develop a solid knowledge base so that better judgments, sizeups, and emergency actions can be decided and implemented. Research in education and training over the years has concluded that lack of knowledge is one of the key reasons why tasks are not performed, are poorly performed, or are performed in a manner that did not achieve the expected results.

Hazardous materials are everywhere in the American society. Homes contain them, as well as businesses, warehouses, places of public assembly, and almost every other type of structure. They can be found in open areas like farm land, wooded areas where clandestine labs operate, and countless other outdoor areas. The first responders must learn to treat fires, collapses, and even traffic accidents as probable hazardous materials incidents. Personal safety at the emergency scene must be the primary focus.

There is a great deal to know and master regarding the nine hazard classes identified and described by the U. S. Department of Transportation (DOT). Paramedics must realize that their safety and the safety of citizens are paramount during the response to a hazardous materials incident. We all know that responder safety is always the first priority during incident operations. This realization is extremely critical when hazardous materials are detected or the preplan suggests that they are present at the incident. Proactive planning can aid the first responder to efficiently and effectively handle critical hazardous materials incidents. One of the most harmful situations is to discover a hazardous material incident well into the response situation. The unexpected often causes undue exposure to harmful substances that can result in immediate and long-term health effects. The first responder and the initial hazardous materials operations crew must have highly developed recognition skills, identification skills, and must know the isolation and protection parameters required for the incident.

Not in the recent history of the EMS has it become so clear that learning is a career-long, life-long requirement that will be the foundation for the demands that lie ahead. We, in EMS, must adopt this principle to move from a tradition-rich past to become truly great providers and protectors available to everyone we serve. We cannot correct the mistakes of the past, but we can use lessons learned to prevent similar mistakes in the future. Knowledge is power. Efficient and effective people are the solution to moving from a good EMS to a truly great one.

Performance Training Systems, Inc. (PTS) has emerged over the past 18 years to become the leading provider of valid testing materials for certification, promotion, and training for fire and emergency medical personnel. More than 35 examination-item banks containing more than 22,000 questions provide the basis for the validated examinations. All products are based on the NFPA Professional Qualifications Standards and selected parts of the DOT National Standard Curriculum for Emergency Medical Technician, Paramedic.

Over the past nine years, PTS has conducted research supporting the development of the Systematic Approach to Examination Preparation® (SAEP). The SAEP has resulted in consistent improvement in scores for persons taking certification, promotion, and training completion examinations. This *Exam Prep* manual is designed to assist paramedics to improve their knowledge, skills, and abilities while seeking training program completion, certification, and promotion. Using the features of SAEP, coupled with helpful examination-taking tips and hints, will help ensure improved performance from a more knowledgeable and skilled paramedic.

The most important factors are that all examination questions used in SAEP were written by paramedics, technical content has been validated through the use of current technical textbooks and other technical reference materials, and job content has been validated by the use of technical review committees representative of the paramedic profession, as well as representatives of training and certification organizations. The examination questions in this *Exam Prep* manual represent an approximate 25 percent sample of the *Paramedic Test-Item Bank* developed and maintained by Performance Training Systems, Inc. These and 33 other test-item banks are being used by 70 fire service certification agencies worldwide, 126 fire academies, and more than 345 fire department training divisions. Forty-six of the fifty state certification agencies use these testing materials in their certification programs.

Purposes of the Emergency Medical Exam Prep Manuals

Performance Training Systems, Inc. provides *Exam Prep* manuals for the following EMS levels:

- Paramedic
- Emergency Medical Technician-Basic
- Medical First Responder

The Emergency Medical *Exam Prep* manuals are designed to provide a random sample of examination items from the major sections of the DOT National Curriculum. Each examination is designed specifically to help you prepare for your National Registry Examination and your local state certification or requalification examination. The *Exam Prep* manuals can also be used in initial training programs and for requalification training.

Since the examination questions have been job-content validated using groups of expert judges from the job incumbent categories, they may also be used for preparing for promotional examinations and for employee selection examinations so long as the pool of job candidates have completed appropriate training and certification in the EMS technical level. The *Exam Prep* manuals are not intended for use in selecting individuals from the general public who have not had appropriate EMS training and certification. Contact Performance Training Systems, Inc., at 800-808-9904, for specific information and procedures on using the *Exam Prep* manuals for employee selection or promotion.

Emergency Medical Service members generally don't like to take examinations. For that matter, few people really like them. The primary purposes of the *Exam Prep* series are to help EMS personnel develop an improved level of knowledge, eliminate examination-taking fear, build self confidence, and develop good study and information mastery skills.

For more information on the number of available test-item banks and the processes of development and validation, visit *medictestbanks.com* or call Performance Training Systems, Inc., toll free, at 800-808-9904.

Introduction to the Systematic Approach to Examination Preparation (SAEP®)

How does SAEP work? SAEP is an organized process of carefully researched phases that permits each person to proceed in examination preparation at that individual's own pace. At certain points, self-study is required to move from one phase of the program to another. Feedback on progress is the basis of SAEP. It is important to follow the program steps carefully to realize the full benefits of the system.

SAEP allows you to prepare for your next comprehensive training, promotional, or certification examination. Just follow the steps to success. Performance Training Systems, Inc., the leader in producing promotional and certification examinations for the fire and emergency medical service industry for over 18 years, has the experience and testing expertise to help you meet your professional goals.

Using the *Exam Prep* manual will enable you to pinpoint areas of weakness in terms of paramedic requirements, and the feedback will provide the reference and page number to help you research the questions that you miss or guess using current technical reference materials. This program is a three-examination set for paramedic as described in the selected parts of the DOT National Standard Curriculum.

Primary benefits of the SAEP in preparing for these examinations include the following:

- Emphasis on areas of weakness
- Immediate feedback
- Saving time and energy
- Learning technical material through context and association
- Helpful examination preparation practices and hints

Phases of SAEP

SAEP is organized in three distinct phases for paramedic as described in portions of the DOT National Standard Curriculum. The phases are briefly described next.

Phase I

This phase includes three examinations containing items that are selected from each major part of the DOT National Standard Curriculum.

An essential part of the SAEP design is to survey your present level of knowledge and build upon it for subsequent examination and self-directed study activities. Therefore, it is suggested that you read the reference materials but do not study or look up any answers while taking the initial examination. Upon completion of the initial examination, you will complete a feedback activity and record examination items that you missed or that you guessed. We ask you to perform certain tasks during the feedback activity. Once you have completed the initial examination and have researched the answers for any questions you missed, you may proceed to the next examination. The process is repeated through and including the third examination in the paramedic series depending on the level of qualification you are seeking.

Phase II

Phase II contains important information about examination-item construction. It provides insight regarding the examination-item developers, how they apply their technology, and hints and tips to help you score higher on any examination. Make sure you read this phase carefully. It is a good practice to read it twice, and study the information a day or two prior to your scheduled examination.

Phase III

Phase III information addresses the mental and physical aspects of examination preparation. By all means, do not skip this part of your preparation. Points can be lost if you are not ready, physically and mentally, for the examination. If you have participated in sporting or other competitive events, you know the importance of this level of preparation. There is no substitute for readiness. Just being able to answer the questions will not move you to a level of excellence and to the top of the examination list for training, promotion, or certification. Quality preparation is much more than just answering examination items.

Supplemental Practice Examination Program

The supplemental practice examination program differs from the SAEP program. It is provided over the Internet 24 hours a day, 7 days a week. This supplemental practice examination allows you to make final preparations immediately before your examination date. You will get an immediate feedback report that includes the questions missed and the references/page numbers for those missed questions. The practice examination will help you concentrate on areas of greatest weakness and will save you time and energy immediately before the examination date. If you choose this method, do not "cram" for the examination. The upcoming helpful hints for examination preparation will explain the reasons for avoiding a "cramming exercise." A supplemental practice examination is available as a part of the cost of this *Exam Prep* book by using the enclosed registration form. Do not forget to fax a copy of your Personal Progress Plotter along with your Registration Form. The data supplied on your Personal Progress Plotter will be kept confidential and will be used by PTS to make future improvements in the *Exam Prep* series. You may take a short practice examination to get the procedure clear in your mind by going to *www.webtesting.cc*.

   Good luck in your efforts to improve your knowledge and skills. Our primary goal is to improve the Emergency Medical Service one person at a time. We want your feedback and impression of the system to help us implement improvements in future editions of the *Exam Prep* series of books. Address your comments and suggestions to *www.medictestbanks.com*.

─────── **Rule 1** ───────

Examination preparation is not easy. Preparation is 95% perspiration and 5% inspiration.

─────── **Rule 2** ───────

Follow the steps very carefully. Do not try to reinvent or shortcut the system. It really works just as it was designed to!

Personal Progress Plotter

Paramedic Exam Prep

Name: _____

Date Started: _____

Date Completed: _____

Paramedic	Number Guessed	Number Missed	Examination Score
Examination I-1			
Examination I-2			
Examination I-3			

Formula to compute Examination Score = ((Number guessed + Number missed) × Point Value per examination item) subtracted from 100.

Note: 150-item examination = .67 points per examination item
200-item examination = .5 points per examination item

Example: In examination I-1 and I-2, 5 examination items were guessed and 8 were missed for a total of 13 on a 150-item examination. The Examination Score would be 100 − (13 × .67 Points) = 91.3

Example: In examination I-3, 5 examination items were guessed and 8 were missed for a total of 13 on a 200-item examination. The Examination Score would be 100 − (13 × .5 Points) = 93.5

Note: To receive your free online practice examination, you must fax a copy of your completed Personal Progress Plotter along with your registration form.

PHASE I

Paramedic

Examination I-1, Beginning DOT National Standard Curriculum for EMT-Paramedic

Examination I-1 contains 150 examination items. Read the reference materials but do not study prior to taking the examination. The examination is designed to identify your weakest areas in terms of selected parts of the DOT National Standard Curriculum. There will be steps in the SAEP that require self-study of specific reference materials. Remove Examination I-1 from the book. Mark all answers in ink. The reason for this is to make sure no changes are made. Do not mark through answers or change answers in any way once you have selected the answer.

Step 1—Take Examination I-1. When you have completed Examination I-1 go to Appendix A and compare your answers with the correct answers. Notice that each answer has reference materials with page numbers. If you missed the correct answer to the examination item, you have a source for conducting your correct answer research.

Step 2—Score Examination I-1. How many examination items did you miss? Write the number of missed examination items in the blank in ink _____. Enter the number of examination items you guessed in this blank _____. Go to your Personal Progress Plotter and enter these numbers in the designated locations.

Step 3—Now the learning begins! Carefully research the page cited in the reference material for the correct answer. For instance, use Mosby, *Paramedic Textbook*, *Revised Second Edition*, go to the page number provided, and find the answer.

Rule 3

Mark with an "X" any examination items for which you guessed the answer. For maximum Return on Effort (ROE) you should also research any answer that you guessed, even if you guessed correctly. Find the correct answer, highlight it, and then read the entire paragraph that contains the answer. Be honest and mark all questions you guessed. Some examinations have a correction for guessing built into the scoring process. The correction for guessing can reduce your final examination score. If you are guessing, you are not mastering the material.

Rule 4

Read questions twice if you have any misunderstanding, especially if the question contains complex directions or activities.

Helpful Hint

Most of the time your first impression is the best. More than 41% of changed answers during our SAEP field test were changed from a right answer to a wrong answer. Another 33% changed their answer from wrong to wrong. Only 26% of changed answers were from wrong to right. In fact, three participants did not make a perfect score of 100% because they changed one right answer to a wrong one! Think twice before you change your answer. The odds are not in your favor.

——————— **Helpful Hint** ———————

Researching correct answers is one of the most important activities in SAEP. Locate the correct answer for all missed examination items. Highlight the correct answer. Then read the entire paragraph containing the answer. This will put the answer in context for you and provide important learning by association.

——————— **Helpful Hint** ———————

Proceed through all missed examination items using the same technique. Reading the entire paragraph improves retention of the information and helps you develop an association with the material and learn the correct answers. This step may sound simple. A major finding during the development and field testing of SAEP was that you learn from your mistakes.

Examination I-1

Directions

Remove Examination I-1 from the manual. First, take a careful look at the examination. There should be 150 examination items. Notice that a blank line precedes each examination-item number. This line is provided for you to enter the answer to the examination item. Write the answer in ink. Remember the rule about changing the answer. Our research has shown that changed answers are often incorrect, and more often than not the answer that is chosen first is correct.

If you guess the answer to a question, place an "X" or a checkmark by your answer. This step is vitally important as you gain and master knowledge. We will explain how we treat the "guessed" items later in SAEP.

Take the examination. Once you complete it, go to Appendix A and score your examination. Once the examination is scored, carefully follow the directions for feedback on the missed and guessed examination items.

_____ **1.** A comprehensive network of coordinated services, including personnel, equipment, and resources established to deliver aid and emergency medical care to the community, is a(n):
A. HMO.
B. EMS system.
C. trauma system.
D. EMD organization.

_____ **2.** The process by which an agency or association grants recognition to an individual who has met its qualifications is:
A. certification.
B. licensure.
C. registration.
D. reciprocity.

_____ **3.** The process by which a governmental agency grants permission to engage in a given occupation to an applicant who has attained the degree of competency required to ensure the public's protection is:
A. certification.
B. licensure.
C. registration.
D. reciprocity.

_____ **4.** The process of entering one's name and essential information within a particular record is:
A. certification.
B. licensure.
C. registration.
D. reciprocity.

_____ **5.** An occupation in which the practitioners have a competence in a specialized body of knowledge or skills that has been recognized by some organization or agency is a:
  A. trade.
  B. craft.
  C. vocation.
  D. profession.

_____ **6.** Which of the following **is not** a physical benefit of achieving acceptable physical fitness?
  A. Decreased blood pressure
  B. Increased oxygen-carrying capacity
  C. Decreased resting heart rate
  D. Decreased metabolism

_____ **7.** Benefits associated with physical fitness include all of the following **except**:
  A. enhanced quality of life.
  B. improved self-image.
  C. enhanced anxiety levels.
  D. maintenance of sound motor skills.

_____ **8.** Which of the following **is not** one of the core elements of physical fitness?
  A. Muscular strength
  B. Cardiovascular endurance
  C. Flexibility
  D. Coordination

_____ **9.** The most common causes of sports injuries include all of the following **except**:
  A. direct trauma.
  B. exsanguination.
  C. fatigue.
  D. exertion.

_____ **10.** The duties of a paramedic set by statutes and regulations are:
  A. ethical responsibilities.
  B. moral responsibilities.
  C. legal responsibilities.
  D. res ipsa loquitur responsibilities.

_____ **11.** Promptly responding to both the physical and emotional needs of every patient is an example of a paramedic's:
  A. ethical responsibilities.
  B. moral responsibilities.
  C. legal responsibilities.
  D. res ipsa loquitur responsibilities.

_____ **12.** If a patient care report is found to be incomplete or inaccurate, the paramedic should:

    A. file a complete new report with the correct information.

    B. add a dated and signed written addendum to the original report.

    C. erase or white out the incorrect information and write in the correct facts.

    D. cross out the incorrect information so that it cannot be read and add the correct information to the bottom of the report, dating it, and signing it.

_____ **13.** The category of law that deals with issues involving conflicts between two or more parties, such as personal injury cases, contract disputes, and matrimonial issues, is:

    A. criminal law.

    B. magistrate law.

    C. civil law.

    D. common law.

_____ **14.** The rules or standards that govern the conduct of members of a particular group or profession are:

    A. morals.

    B. prerequisites.

    C. ethics.

    D. codes.

_____ **15.** The process in which the size of a cell decreases as a result of a decreasing workload is known as:

    A. atrophy.

    B. hypertrophy.

    C. hyperplasia.

    D. metaplasia.

_____ **16.** The process in which one type of cell is replaced by another type of cell **not** normal for that tissue is known as:

    A. atrophy.

    B. hypertrophy.

    C. hyperplasia.

    D. metaplasia.

_____ **17.** The process in which an increase in the number of cells results from an increasing workload is known as:

    A. atrophy.

    B. hypertrophy.

    C. hyperplasia.

    D. metaplasia.

_____ **18.** The process that produces an increase in cell size as a result of increasing workload is known as:

    A. atrophy.

    B. hypertrophy.

    C. hyperplasia.

    D. metaplasia.

_____ **19.** A change in cell size, shape, or appearance caused by an external stressor is known as:
   A. mitosis.
   B. dysplasia.
   C. dilation.
   D. catabolism.

_____ **20.** Which of the following is an official name of this common sedative?
   A. Valium
   B. 7-chloro-1, 3-dihydro-1-methyl-5-phenyl-2H-1, 4-benzodiazepin-2-one
   C. Diazepam
   D. Diazepam, USP

_____ **21.** Which of the following is a generic name?
   A. Ethyl 1-methyl-4-phenylisonipecotate hydrochloride
   B. Meperidine hydrochloride
   C. Demerol hydrochloride
   D. Meperidine hydrochloride, USP

_____ **22.** Which of the following **is not** one of the four main sources of drugs?
   A. Plants
   B. Minerals
   C. Petroleum
   D. Animals

_____ **23.** The correct agent and action for the control of CHF and pulmonary edema is:
   A. nitroglycerine, with a reduction of afterload via arterial smooth muscle relaxation.
   B. furosemide, with a reduction of circulating volume.
   C. reserpine (Serpalan), with a reduction of circulating norepinephrine.
   D. labetalol (Normodyne), with a combined reduction of alpha and beta effects.

_____ **24.** The official standard for information about pharmaceuticals is the:
   A. Federal Drug Administration (FDA).
   B. United States Adopted Name Council (USANC).
   C. United States Pharmacopoeia (USP)
   D. Federal Pharmacological Agency (FPA)

_____ **25.** All of the following are Schedule I drugs **except**:
   A. heroin.
   B. LSD.
   C. opium.
   D. mescaline.

_____ **26.** Under the tongue, between the cheek and gums, the eyes, the nose, and the ear and ear canal are sites where medications can be absorbed into the body through the:
   A. arterioles.
   B. capillaries.
   C. venules.
   D. mucous membranes.

_____ **27.** <u>Scenario</u>: A physician orders 225 mg of acetaminophen to a pediatric patient. The liquid acetaminophen is packaged in a concentration of 160 mg in 5 ml of solution. The amount of medication you would administer is:
A. 6 ml.
B. 7 ml.
C. 8 ml.
D. 9 ml.

_____ **28.** <u>Scenario</u>: A physician orders .25 mg/kg of Cardizem for a patient who weighs 176 pounds. The concentration of Cardizem is 25 mg in 5 ml. The amount of medication that you would administer is:
A. 18 ml
B. 20 ml
C. 23 ml
D. 28 ml

_____ **29.** <u>Scenario</u>: A physician orders administration of heparin at 1000 units per hour to a patient. You have on hand 25,000 units of heparin in 500 cc of normal saline. You will use a microdrip set to run this IV infusion. What should the infusion rate be?
A. 16 gtts/minute
B. 18 gtts/minute
C. 20 gtts/minute
D. 22 gtts/minute

_____ **30.** <u>Scenario</u>: A physician orders D5½ normal saline at 125 cc/hour. The administration tubing is a macrodrip set with a drip factor of 10 gtts/ml. At what drip rate would you run the infusion?
A. 18.8 gtts/minute
B. 20.8 gtts/minute
C. 26.8 gtts/minute
D. 30.8 gtts/minute

_____ **31.** A milliliter equals:
A. 1/10 of a liter.
B. 1/100 of a liter.
C. 1/1000 of a liter.
D. 1/10,000 of a liter.

_____ **32.** The exchange of common symbols is:
A. speaking.
B. listening.
C. communication.
D. understanding.

_____ **33.** In EMS, failure to communicate effectively may be the result of all of the following <u>except</u>:
A. prejudice.
B. lack of privacy.
C. external distractions.
D. feelings of empathy towards the patient.

_____ **34.** By 4 to 6 months, a child should have:
   A. increased birth weight, but in no set pattern.
   B. doubled his or her birth weight.
   C. tripled his or her birth weight.
   D. quadrupled his or her birth weight.

_____ **35.** All of the following are advantages of assisted-living facilities for older adults compared to home-care or nursing-home facilities **except** a greater sense of:
   A. financial dependence.
   B. privacy.
   C. control.
   D. independence.

_____ **36.** Causes of increased carbon dioxide production include all of the following **except**:
   A. fever.
   B. hyperventilation.
   C. shivering.
   D. muscle exertion.

_____ **37.** Without adequate airway maintenance and ventilation, the patient can succumb to brain injury or death in how many minutes?
   A. 2-4 minutes
   B. 4-6 minutes
   C. 6-10 minutes
   D. 10-12 minutes

_____ **38.** Manual maneuvers used to open a patient's airway:
   A. are contraindicated in most patients outside of the emergency department.
   B. are difficult to perform for even the most experienced prehospital providers.
   C. are often neglected in the prehospital setting.
   D. don't usually work without more extensive airway maintenance.

_____ **39.** Cartilage that separates the right and left nasal cavities is the:
   A. larynx.
   B. epiglottis.
   C. inferior turbinates.
   D. septum.

_____ **40.** All of the following are pairs of sinuses **except** the:
   A. oropharyngeal sinuses.
   B. ethmoid sinuses.
   C. frontal sinuses.
   D. sphenoid sinuses.

_____ **41.** Oxygen concentrations in the blood can be affected by:
   A. decreased hemoglobin concentration.
   B. pulmonary edema.
   C. ventilation/perfusion mismatch.
   D. All of the above.

_____ **42.** When using the end-tidal carbon dioxide detector as a tool to determine if endotracheal intubation has been correctly obtained, the absence of carbon dioxide in exhaled air indicates the endotracheal tube has been:
A. correctly placed.
B. placed in the esophagus.
C. placed in the right mainstem bronchus.
D. placed in the left mainstem bronchus.

_____ **43.** The hypoxic drive is regulated by:
A. PaO_2 levels.
B. $PaCO_2$ levels.
C. high oxygen saturation percentage.
D. low oxygen saturation percentage.

_____ **44.** The airflow during a **maximum** exhalation is the:
A. peak expiratory flow.
B. tidal volume.
C. tidal reserve.
D. functional residual capacity.

_____ **45.** Air enters the nasal cavity through the:
A. esophagus.
B. external nares.
C. glottic opening.
D. trachea.

_____ **46.** One of the **best** techniques for establishing patient rapport when taking a history is to:
A. speak loudly and establish your authority with the patient.
B. use specific medical terms when asking questions of the patient.
C. establish eye contact and greet the patient by name or surname.
D. advance toward the patient and begin your physical exam.

_____ **47.** The technique of _____ involves careful, informed visual observation.
A. auscultation
B. inspection
C. palpation
D. percussion

_____ **48.** Physical exam techniques include all of the following **except**:
A. inspection.
B. palpation.
C. auscultation.
D. association.

_____ **49.** Which technique does a paramedic use to effectively evaluate for tenderness, rigidity, pain, or crepitus?
A. Palpation
B. Auscultation
C. Percussion
D. Inspection

_____ **50.** The process in which a paramedic places a hand on a body part and then sharply taps a distal knuckle with the tip of another finger is known as:
  A. hyperresonance.
  B. palpation.
  C. percussion.
  D. observation.

_____ **51.** <u>Scenario</u>: You are sent to the home of an insulin-dependent diabetic female. You ask her to state her name, the month, and her address. This would be an example of:
  A. assessing memory and attention.
  B. interrogation.
  C. assessing mood.
  D. assessing judgment.

_____ **52.** As part of the mental status exam, assessing a patient's mood can be accomplished by:
  A. observing verbal and nonverbal behavior.
  B. determining coherence of thoughts.
  C. listening to the articulation of words.
  D. observing personal hygiene.

_____ **53.** A paramedic should use _____ to recognize potential hazards at the scene of an emergency.
  A. sight and smell
  B. taste
  C. touch and hearing
  D. all senses

_____ **54.** <u>Scenario</u>: You are responding to a collision between a car and a truck. Prior to arrival, you consider _____ as a potential hazard at this scene.
  A. fire and traffic only
  B. broken glass and chemical spills
  C. leaking gas and downed electrical wires
  D. All of the above.

_____ **55.** Always use a properly fitted HEPA mask when managing a patient you suspect has:
  A. influenza.
  B. TB.
  C. COPD.
  D. asthma.

_____ **56.** <u>Scenario</u>: You respond to shots fired, man down. You should enter the scene when:
  A. you observe the gunman fleeing the scene.
  B. you get to the location.
  C. dispatch informs you the scene is safe.
  D. police officers arrive and secure the scene.

_____ **57.** The proper procedure for gaining access to a patient at the scene of a domestic violence incident would be to:
   A. have your partner distract the assailant.
   B. wait for law enforcement personnel to arrive.
   C. have your dispatcher tell the patient to come outside.
   D. leave the scene and become available for the next assignment.

_____ **58.** Who or what is usually the **best** source of information about the nature of your patient's illness if he is alert and oriented?
   A. Visual cues
   B. Diagnostic tests
   C. The patient himself
   D. Family members and bystanders

_____ **59.** Paramedics are able to treat patients with the same techniques as other clinicians with the **exception** that they:
   A. are far less trained than other practitioners.
   B. perform these procedures in uncontrollable and unpredictable environments.
   C. treat life-threatening emergencies only.
   D. are not allowed to make independent decisions.

_____ **60.** The term _acuity_ refers to:
   A. the severity of the patient's condition.
   B. the use of standing orders for care.
   C. the use of an algorithm.
   D. critical thinking and decision-making skills.

_____ **61.** Upon arrival at the hospital, you typically would communicate all of the following to the emergency department staff **except** the:
   A. mechanism of injury.
   B. assessment findings.
   C. patient's health insurance information.
   D. interventions provided along with patient response.

_____ **62.** The **most** important reason to maintain open lines of communication with other heath care providers is to:
   A. ensure the continuity of care upon arrival at the ED.
   B. prevent the ED staff from having to find you and ask additional questions.
   C. promote a good working relationship with the ED staff.
   D. ensure that you are following company/institution policy.

_____ **63.** _____ is the key link in the chain that results in the best possible patient outcome.
   A. Coordination
   B. Communication
   C. Confrontation
   D. Conceptualization

_____ **64.** Your prehospital care report's accuracy is affected by all of the following **except**:
   A. proper spelling.
   B. approved abbreviations.
   C. paramedic opinion.
   D. proper acronyms.

_____ **65.** The only truly factual record of the events on an EMS call is the:
   A. communications center report.
   B. emergency department chart.
   C. prehospital care report.
   D. medical control report.

_____ **66.** The prehospital care report should document all of the following **except**:
   A. treatments provided.
   B. subjective opinions.
   C. pertinent negatives.
   D. objective observations.

_____ **67.** Use of prehospital care reports for quality improvement is an example of their _____ use.
   A. administrative
   B. legal
   C. medical
   D. patient care

_____ **68.** Ninety-seven percent of all trauma-related vascular injuries result from:
   A. blast-related injuries.
   B. compression injuries.
   C. penetration trauma.
   D. post-traumatic hypertension.

_____ **69.** In an underwater detonation, the lethal range for the charge **increases**:
   A. threefold.
   B. fourfold.
   C. fivefold.
   D. sixfold.

_____ **70.** The projectiles that are thrown during an explosion create numerous injuries. Among these injuries are:
   A. overpressure injuries.
   B. underpressure injuries.
   C. impaled object injuries.
   D. entrapment injuries.

_____ **71.** During the tertiary phase of a blast, **most** injuries are associated with:
   A. overpressure.
   B. heat exposure.
   C. projectiles.
   D. entrapment.

_____ **72.** The transition between normal function and death is called:
   A. homeostasis.
   B. hemorrhage.
   C. exsanguination.
   D. shock.

_____ **73.** The part of the nervous system that speeds up the heart rate is the:
   A. parasympathetic nervous system.
   B. autonomic nervous system.
   C. sympathetic nervous system.
   D. central nervous system.

_____ **74.** The vessels that distribute blood to the organs and operate under high pressure are called:
   A. leukocytes.
   B. capillaries.
   C. veins.
   D. arteries.

_____ **75.** The **most** **common** form of trauma is:
   A. fractures.
   B. penetrating wounds.
   C. blunt trauma.
   D. soft tissue injuries.

_____ **76.** The layer of skin that contains adipose/fat tissue is the:
   A. epidermis.
   B. dermis.
   C. subcutaneous.
   D. fascia.

_____ **77.** How does the integumentary system prevent pathogens from attacking the body?
   A. Leukocytes in the skin attack pathogens.
   B. Antibodies in the skin attack pathogens.
   C. Skin provides a pathway out of the body for pathogens.
   D. Skin provides a protective barrier against pathogens.

_____ **78.** The layer of the skin that contains nerve endings is the:
   A. fascia.
   B. epidermis.
   C. subcutaneous.
   D. dermis.

_____ **79.** The **second** leading cause of death in children under the age of 12 is:
   A. cardiac arrest.
   B. automobile accidents.
   C. burns.
   D. drowning.

_____ 80. The body's response to burns occurs in stages. In this stage there is a pain response and an outpouring of catecholamines. The patient displays tachycardia, tachypnea, mild hypertension, and mild anxiety. This phase is called the _____ phase.
A. resolution
B. hypermetabolic
C. fluid shift
D. emergent

_____ 81. The area of the body that accounts for **most** deaths in auto accidents is the:
A. spine.
B. chest.
C. head.
D. pelvis.

_____ 82. Which of the following facial injuries would be **least threatening** to the patient's life?
A. La Fort II fracture
B. Fracture of nasal septum and cartilage
C. Fractured zygoma
D. Mandibular fracture

_____ 83. A patient sustains significant head trauma. A fracture of which of the following bones poses the **greatest** potential for concurrent nerve/brain injury?
A. Lacrimal bone
B. Mastoid process
C. Maxillary bone
D. Cribriform plate

_____ 84. In falls, which section of the spinal column is the **most** prone to compression injury?
A. Cervical
B. Thoracic
C. Lumbar
D. Sacral

_____ 85. Which of the following is the **most prominent** mechanism of injury associated with spinal cord injuries?
A. Falls
B. Auto accidents
C. Penetrating injuries
D. Sports-related injuries

_____ 86. The central nervous system is made up of the:
A. brain and meninges.
B. brain and cervical spinal column.
C. brain and spinal cord.
D. spinal cord only.

_____ **87.** <u>Scenario</u>: You are dispatched to a motor vehicle accident. On arrival you notice that the car struck a parked vehicle at approximately 55 mph. Your 24-year-old female patient is complaining of difficulty breathing. Breath sounds are diminished bilaterally. The patient tells you that at the last minute she recognized the impending accident and held her breath. You expect the paper-bag syndrome, which involves the rupture of:
    A. arteries.
    B. intestines.
    C. the spleen.
    D. alveoli.

_____ **88.** In automobile collisions, the type of impact **<u>most</u> <u>commonly</u>** associated with aortic rupture is:
    A. lateral.
    B. frontal.
    C. rollover.
    D. rotational.

_____ **89.** Which of the following statements regarding the mortality of thoracic injuries is **<u>correct</u>**?
    A. A majority of these deaths are secondary to injury to the respiratory tree.
    B. A majority of these deaths are secondary to injury to the heart and great vessels.
    C. A majority of these deaths are secondary to injury to the brain and great vessels.
    D. A majority of these deaths are primarily due to external thoracic trauma, such as ecchymosis or lacerations.

_____ **90.** Currently, the **<u>number</u>-<u>one</u>** traumatic cause of mortality and morbidity is:
    A. penetrating trauma.
    B. motor vehicle accidents.
    C. falls.
    D. blast injuries.

_____ **91.** Which of the following statements about abdominal injuries **<u>is</u> <u>true</u>**?
    A. Signs and symptoms associated with abdominal injuries take time to develop.
    B. External bleeding is the best indicator of severity in abdominal trauma.
    C. Trauma to the thoracic cavity does not cause abdominal injuries.
    D. Cavitation follows low-velocity penetration.

_____ **92.** The **<u>greatest</u>** single cause of musculoskeletal injuries in the United States is:
    A. falls.
    B. gunshot wounds.
    C. motor vehicle accidents.
    D. sporting injuries.

_____ **93.** The musculoskeletal system is a complex arrangement of levers and fulcrums providing motion and support for the body. All of the following are functions of the musculoskeletal system **except**:
  A. glycogen storage.
  B. protecting vital organs.
  C. production of blood cells.
  D. essential salt storage.

_____ **94.** When EMS is called to the scene of a non-life-threatening injury, it is important for the medical provider to keep in mind that:
  A. displaying a concerned attitude and a professional demeanor may reinforce the patient's behavior of dialing 911, and must be avoided.
  B. while the EMS provider sees patients with all types of injuries and illnesses ranging from benign to severe, the patient may be uncomfortable in this environment and should be supported emotionally, as well as physically.
  C. EMS is seldom activated for non-life-threats and therefore the provider should not be concerned with the treatment of simple injuries.
  D. the application of the cardiac monitor allows the provider to bill for advanced care.

_____ **95.** Minute blood vessels, surrounded by layers of salts deposited in collagen fibers, travel lengthwise along the bone through small tubes known as:
  A. perforating canals.
  B. osteocytic pores.
  C. haversian canals.
  D. osteoblastic pores.

_____ **96.** All of the following comprise the upper airway **except** the:
  A. larynx.
  B. nasal cavity.
  C. pharynx.
  D. trachea.

_____ **97.** The **most** **superior** portion of the pharynx is the:
  A. hypopharynx.
  B. laryngopharynx.
  C. nasopharynx.
  D. oropharynx.

_____ **98.** The vocal cords and the space between them are referred to as the:
  A. arytenoids.
  B. false vocal cords.
  C. glottic opening.
  D. vestibule.

_____ **99.** When swallowing, the structure that occludes the trachea to prevent food from passing into the trachea is the:
  A. carina.
  B. epiglottis.
  C. uvula.
  D. vallecula.

_____**100.** Which device, when inserted improperly, may advance too far and lodge in the right mainstem bronchus?
   A. Endotracheal tube
   B. Esophageal gastric tracheal airway
   C. Esophageal obturator airway
   D. Oropharyngeal airway

_____**101.** Approximately _____ percent of Americans who have coronary heart disease die before ever reaching the hospital.
   A. 25
   B. 50
   C. 75
   D. 80

_____**102.** Which of the following **is** **not** considered a modifiable risk factor for coronary heart disease?
   A. Diet
   B. Gender
   C. Obesity
   D. Psychosocial tension

_____**103.** Which of the following **is** **not** a risk factor of cardiovascular disease?
   A. Heredity
   B. Hypercholesterolemia
   C. Cocaine use
   D. Macular degeneration

_____**104.** The base of the heart lies at the level of the:
   A. 1st rib.
   B. 2nd rib.
   C. 3rd rib.
   D. 4th rib.

_____**105.** The thick middle tissue layer of the heart is the:
   A. endocardium.
   B. epicardium.
   C. myocardium.
   D. pericardium.

_____**106.** Which of the following **is** **not** a main part of the aorta?
   A. Abdominal
   B. Ascending
   C. Descending
   D. Thoracic

_____**107.** The component of blood vessels that consists of elastic fiber and muscle is the:
   A. lumen.
   B. tunica adventitia.
   C. tunica intima.
   D. tunica media.

_____**108.** Poiseuille's Law states that blood flow through a vessel is:
    A. directly proportional to the fourth power of the vessel's radius.
    B. directly proportional to the vessel's radius.
    C. directly proportional to the vessel's length to the fourth power.
    D. indirectly proportional to the vessel's radius.

_____**109.** The amount of blood ejected by the heart in one cardiac contraction is known as:
    A. cardiac cycle.
    B. cardiac output.
    C. ejection fraction.
    D. stroke volume.

_____**110.** The pressure in the ventricle at the end of diastole is known as:
    A. afterload.
    B. ejection fraction.
    C. end-systole volume.
    D. preload.

_____**111.** The **best** mathematical means to understand blood pressure is:
    A. blood pressure = (cardiac output × heart rate) × systemic vascular resistance.
    B. blood pressure = heart rate × vascular resistance.
    C. blood pressure = (heart rate × vascular resistance) − ejection fraction.
    D. blood pressure = (stroke volume × heart rate) × peripheral vascular resistance.

_____**112.** During systole, which of the following valves is open?
    A. Semilunar
    B. Bicuspid
    C. Mitral
    D. Tricuspid

_____**113.** The interval from the end of one cardiac contraction to the end of the next is known as:
    A. the cardiac cycle.
    B. diastole.
    C. the heart beat.
    D. systole.

_____**114.** Increased venous return to the heart results in greater preload and thus:
    A. greater afterload.
    B. greater stroke volume.
    C. lesser stroke volume.
    D. less myocardial stretch.

_____**115.** Which of the following **is not** an appropriate management for a patient with a general complaint of feeling weak and dizzy?
    A. Assist ventilations with bag-valve-mask.
    B. Consider the administration of promethazine.
    C. Evaluate blood glucose level.
    D. Monitor cardiac rhythm.

_____ **116.** The _____ nervous system extends throughout the body and is comprised of the cranial nerves arising from the brain and the peripheral nerves arising from the spinal cord.
  A. afferent
  B. efferent
  C. peripheral
  D. somatic

_____ **117.** The _____ nervous system is responsible for controlling vegetative functions including decreased heart rate and bronchiole constriction, as well as digestion and defecation.
  A. afferent
  B. parasympathetic
  C. somatic
  D. sympathetic

_____ **118.** The portion of the nerve cell that conducts impulses away from the soma/cell body is the:
  A. axon.
  B. dendrite.
  C. neurotransmitter.
  D. synaptic terminal.

_____ **119.** The neurotransmitter found in the synaptic terminals of the sympathetic nerves is:
  A. acetylcholine.
  B. adrenaline.
  C. dopamine.
  D. norepinephrine.

_____ **120.** The tough outermost layer of the meninges is the:
  A. arachnoid membrane.
  B. cerebellum.
  C. dura mater.
  D. pia mater.

_____ **121.** Which of the following disorders has the **highest** mortality rate?
  A. Diabetic ketoacidosis
  B. Hyperglycemic hyperosmolar nonketotic coma
  C. Hypoglycemia
  D. Insulin shock

_____ **122.** A chemical substance released by a gland that controls or affects processes in other glands or body systems is:
  A. a hormone.
  B. dopamine.
  C. a neurotransmitter.
  D. seratonin.

_____**123.** Which of the following is an exocrine gland?
  A. Adrenal gland
  B. Pancreas
  C. Pineal gland
  D. Salivary gland

_____**124.** An exaggerated response by the immune system to a foreign substance is:
  A. an allergic reaction.
  B. an allergy.
  C. hypersensitivity.
  D. an immune response.

_____**125.** A life-threatening emergency that occurs due to an unusually exaggerated allergic reaction to a foreign protein or other substance is:
  A. anaphylaxis.
  B. hypersensitivity.
  C. an immune response.
  D. a primary response.

_____**126.** What percentage of emergency department visits are due to gastrointestinal emergencies?
  A. 5 percent
  B. 10 percent
  C. 15 percent
  D. 20 percent

_____**127.** All of the following are considered predisposing or risk factors for upper GI bleeding **except**:
  A. atherosclerosis.
  B. diabetes.
  C. hemorrhoids.
  D. hypertension.

_____**128.** All of the following structures are part of the lower gastrointestinal tract **except** the:
  A. duodenum.
  B. ileum.
  C. jejunum.
  D. large intestine.

_____**129.** A sharp, localized pain that originates in walls of the body such as skeletal muscles is:
  A. parietal pain.
  B. referred pain.
  C. somatic pain.
  D. visceral pain.

_____**130.** The leading cause of end-stage renal disease is:
  A. hepatitis.
  B. kidney infections.
  C. renal calculi.
  D. uncontrolled diabetes mellitus.

_____ **131.** All of the following are major functions of the urinary system **except**:
  A. controlling the development of erythrocytes.
  B. ensuring that glucose is eliminated.
  C. maintaining pH balance.
  D. removing toxic wastes.

_____ **132.** When patients are inside a burning building, they inhale the products of incomplete combustion. The carbon monoxide displaces oxygen because its affinity for binding to hemoglobin is _____ times **greater** **than** that of oxygen.
  A. 200
  B. 150
  C. 100
  D. 50

_____ **133.** Scenario: A patient was mixing pesticides to spray in his garden and suddenly began experiencing excessive salivation, abdominal pain, and dizziness. The **most** **likely** route of toxic exposure is:
  A. absorption.
  B. ingestion.
  C. inhalation.
  D. injection.

_____ **134.** Fifty percent of accidental poisonings occur in patients aged:
  A. 0-6 years.
  B. 7-18 years.
  C. 18-25 years.
  D. 25-44 years.

_____ **135.** Which component of the hematopoietic system is responsible for removing thrombocytes and erythrocytes?
  A. Bone marrow
  B. Kidneys
  C. Liver
  D. Spleen

_____ **136.** All of the following are compensatory mechanisms of the hematopoietic system to conserve blood volume **except**:
  A. decreased chronotropic effects.
  B. increased inotropic effects.
  C. tachycardia.
  D. vasoconstriction.

_____ **137.** A medical condition caused or exacerbated by the weather, terrain, atmospheric pressure, or other local features is an:
  A. environmental emergency.
  B. environmental homeostasis.
  C. unbalanced homeostasis.
  D. untoward event.

_____**138.** A significantly increased incidence of mortality occurs when the body core temperature is <u>less</u> <u>than</u>:

    A. 95°F.

    B. 90°F.

    C. 88°F.

    D. 86°F.

_____**139.** All of the following are considered risk factors for developing an environmental illness <u>except</u>:

    A. diabetes.

    B. emphysema.

    C. hyperactivity.

    D. very young children.

_____**140.** All of the following environmental factors will exacerbate a preexisting illness <u>except</u>:

    A. acute changes in temperature.

    B. high atmospheric pressures.

    C. humidity.

    D. seasonal allergens.

_____**141.** The _____ is a major component of the lymphatic system.

    A. gall bladder

    B. liver

    C. pancreas

    D. spleen

_____**142.** _____ are microorganisms that reside in the body without ordinarily causing disease.

    A. Normal flora

    B. Opportunistic pathogens

    C. Pathogens

    D. Virulent parasites

_____**143.** Which agency is considered a public health agency?

    A. CDC

    B. FEMA

    C. NFPA

    D. USFPA

_____**144.** _____ is a person's observable conduct and activity.

    A. Affect

    B. Attitude

    C. Behavior

    D. Rapport

_____**145.** A situation in which a person's behavior is so unusual that it alarms another person or requires intervention is:

    A. a behavioral emergency.

    B. a critical affective period.

    C. an emotional dilemma.

    D. a psychological crisis.

_____**146.** The relative shortness of the _____ structure and its proximity to the vaginal canal enable bacteria to enter the bladder easily.
   A. hymen
   B. perineum
   C. urethra
   D. vestibule

_____**147.** Pregnancy affects cardiac status by:
   A. reducing the mother's circulating volume by 45 percent.
   B. increasing the maternal heart rate by 25-30 beats per minute.
   C. decreasing maternal cardiac output by 40 percent.
   D. increasing the maternal circulating volume by 45 percent.

_____**148.** Airbags have been introduced to help reduce the injuries received in automobile collisions. With certain age groups, airbags have inflicted serious injury or death. The age group that is **most** susceptible to these injuries is:
   A. geriatric.
   B. pediatric.
   C. adult.
   D. adolescent.

_____**149.** Falls are a common mechanism of injury in geriatric patients. In these cases, the force required to break a bone is **generally**:
   A. much greater than in other patients.
   B. the same as in other patients.
   C. slightly greater than in other patients.
   D. less than in other patients.

_____**150.** What impact is the geriatric population expected to have on the frequency of EMS calls over the next several years?
   A. Moderate decrease
   B. Significant decrease
   C. Significant increase
   D. Relative stability

Did you score higher than 80 percent on Examination I-1? Circle Yes or No in ink. (We will return to your answer to this question later in SAEP.)

   Now that you have finished the Feedback Step for Examination I-1, it is time to repeat the process by taking another comprehensive examination of the *DOT, Paramedic National Standard Curriculum.*

Examination I-2, Adding Difficulty and Depth

During Examination I-2 progress will be made in developing depth of knowledge and skills.

Step 1—Take Examination I-2. When you have completed Examination I-2, go to Appendix A and compare your answers with the correct answers.

Step 2—Score Examination I-2. How many examination items did you miss? Write the number of missed examination items in the blank in ink _____ . Enter the number of examination items you guessed in this blank _____. Enter these numbers in the designated locations on your Personal Progress Plotter.

Step 3—Once again, the learning begins. During the feedback step, research the correct answer using Appendix A information for Examination I-2. Highlight the correct answer during your research of the reference materials. Read the entire paragraph containing the correct answer.

——— **Helpful Hint** ———

Follow each step carefully to realize the best Return on Effort (ROE). Would you consider investing your money in a venture without some chance of return on that investment? Examination preparation is no different. You are investing time expecting a significant return for that time. If, indeed, time is money, then you are investing money and are due a return on that investment. Doing things right and doing the right things in examination preparation will ensure the maximum return on effort.

Examination I-2

Directions

Remove Examination I-2 from the manual. First, take a careful look at the examination. There should be 150 examination items. Notice that a blank line precedes each examination-item number. This line is provided for you to enter the answer to the examination item. Write the answer in ink. Remember the rule about not changing your answers. Our research shows that changed answers are most often changed to an incorrect answer, and, more often than not, the answer that is chosen first is correct.

If you guess an answer, place an "X" or a check mark by your answer. This step is vitally important to gain and master knowledge. We will explain how we treat the "guessed" items later in SAEP.

Take the examination. Once you complete it, go to Appendix A and score your examination. After the examination is scored, carefully follow the directions for feedback of the missed and guessed examination items.

_____ **1.** Many traditional EMS treatments and practices have been abandoned or refined as a result of:
 A. lawsuits.
 B. research.
 C. court orders.
 D. legislation.

_____ **2.** One result of the increasing specialization of health care facilities has been expansion of the paramedic role in:
 A. neonatal care.
 B. BCLS.
 C. critical care transport.
 D. ACLS.

_____ **3.** Paramedics working in close contact with medical direction to provide care to patients in their homes and to treat patients at emergency scenes without transport are examples of the expanded scope of practice in:
 A. managed care.
 B. primary care.
 C. tertiary care.
 D. dependent care.

_____ **4.** Safety inspections, accident prevention programs, medical screenings, and vaccination and immunization programs are some of the responsibilities of paramedics working in:
 A. sports medicine.
 B. neonatal intensive care programs.
 C. ACLS.
 D. industrial medicine.

_____ **5.** Many professional sports teams have found paramedics to be effective complements to their:

    A. HMOs.

    B. physician assistants.

    C. players.

    D. trainers.

_____ **6.** Shift work and loud pagers are two common stressors in EMS work that fall into the category of:

    A. administrative.

    B. emotional.

    C. physical.

    D. scene related.

_____ **7.** <u>Scenario</u>: Your EMS partner has been through some hard times lately. He broke up with his wife a couple of months ago, and his father died last month. After not smoking for years, he's taken it up again and chain smokes now. He's sometimes rude to patients, and when you try to talk with him about this, he cuts you off. Your partner is probably using stress management techniques that are described as:

    A. administrative/active.

    B. synergistic.

    C. beneficial.

    D. detrimental/negative.

_____ **8.** The stress management technique of controlled breathing works by:

    A. reducing adrenaline levels.

    B. increasing blood pressure.

    C. increasing ACTH levels.

    D. speeding digestion.

_____ **9.** Items that paramedics can document on patient forms to help implement future injury prevention programs **include**:

    A. scene conditions at the time of EMS arrival.

    B. risks that EMS personnel had to overcome.

    C. use or non-use of protective devices.

    D. All of the above.

_____ **10.** <u>Scenario</u>: A patient who has no other signs and symptoms of medical problems, has been treated by paramedics for a sprained wrist, and is being transported in a non-emergency mode suffers a stroke while in the ambulance. What do you think would be the <u>likely</u> outcome of a negligence lawsuit brought by the patient?

    A. The suit would succeed because four elements of negligence were present.

    B. The suit would fail because the plaintiff could not demonstrate that the paramedics' actions were the proximate cause of the stroke.

    C. The suit would fail because the plaintiff failed to demonstrate malice on the part of the plaintiffs.

    D. The suit would succeed because the paramedics had a duty to act and the patient suffered actual damages.

_____ **11.** Which of the following is a recommended procedure for paramedics treating a patient at a crime scene?
  A. Focus on the patient's needs rather than the possible evidence.
  B. Leave holes in a patient's clothing made by bullets or knives intact if possible.
  C. If you had to move anything, tell law enforcement officers in a phone or radio report after you have transferred patient care at the hospital.
  D. All of the above.

_____ **12.** A paramedic may be responsible for the negligence of EMT-Bs and EMT-Is under his supervision under the:
  A. res ipsa loquitur clause.
  B. elastic clause.
  C. ex parte Milligan decision.
  D. borrowed servant doctrine.

_____ **13.** An off-duty paramedic who provides advanced life support skills at an emergency scene:
  A. is protected by Good Samaritan laws in all states.
  B. is assumed to provide a proximate cause for a negligence charge.
  C. may be charged with practicing medicine without a license.
  D. shares liability with the medical director of his EMS system.

_____ **14.** State laws requiring the reporting of births, deaths, certain infectious diseases, and child and elder abuse and neglect may require the paramedic to breach the obligation to protect the patient's:
  A. autonomy.
  B. confidentiality.
  C. well-being.
  D. refusal of consent.

_____ **15.** As blood volume is lost due to a traumatic injury, the body's response is to:
  A. increase heart rate and decrease systemic vascular resistance.
  B. decrease heart rate and vasoconstrict major veins.
  C. increase heart rate and bronchodilation.
  D. decrease heart rate and promote peripheral vasoconstriction.

_____ **16.** A common cause of damage in primary multiple organ dysfunction syndrome is:
  A. neuroendocrine response.
  B. vasodilation and clotting abnormalities.
  C. damage to endothelium of the vasculature.
  D. inadequate perfusion from a traumatic incident.

_____ **17.** Which of the following **is not** part of the body's response in secondary MODS?
  A. Catecholamine release is inhibited.
  B. Inflammatory mediators enter the system.
  C. Plasma protein systems are activated.
  D. Release of endorphins contributes to vasodilation.

_____ **18.** The <u>final</u> common pathway of multiple organ dysfunction syndrome is:
   A. impairment of two or more organ systems.
   B. hypoxemia and hypocapnia.
   C. hyperperfusion.
   D. inflammatory response.

_____ **19.** Which of the following <u>is not</u> one of the body's three chief lines of defense against infection and injury?
   A. Anatomic barriers
   B. Psychosomatic shields
   C. Inflammatory response
   D. Immune response

_____ **20.** Organophosphate poisoning can be treated with IV administration of atropine. Symptoms of organophosphate poisoning include all of the following <u>except</u>:
   A. emesis.
   B. hypotension.
   C. tachycardia.
   D. salivation.

_____ **21.** In lieu of conduction disturbances, if the heart's dominant pacemaker fails to generate an impulse, next, an impulse will be generated at a slower rate by the:
   A. Purkinje network.
   B. sinoatrial (SA) node.
   C. atrioventricular (AV) node.
   D. bundle branches.

_____ **22.** The ability of the heart to self-generate electrical impulses is known as:
   A. conduction velocity.
   B. contractility.
   C. automaticity.
   D. inotropism.

_____ **23.** The <u>primary</u> ions involved in action potential synthesis and transmission are:
   A. K^+, Na^+, Hg^{+++}.
   B. Na^+, K^+.
   C. Ca^{++}, Na^+.
   D. Ca^{++}, H^+

_____ **24.** What is the drug of choice for a patient suffering from grand mal seizures?
   A. Romazicon
   B. Valproic acid
   C. Dilantin
   D. Ethosuximide

_____ **25.** Calcium channel blockers such as verapamil (Calan) and diltiazem (Cardizem) will have what cardiovascular effect?
   A. Decrease PVR, widen QRS, increase afterload
   B. Increase PVR, widen QRS, increase afterload
   C. Decrease SA and AV node automaticity; decrease conductivity through the AV node
   D. Prolong the QT interval

_____ **26.** All of the following reduce the risk of accidental needle sticks **except**:
   A. minimizing the tasks performed in the back of a moving ambulance.
   B. dropping sharps on the floor for disposal after the ambulance has stopped.
   C. disposing of used sharps in a sharps container.
   D. recapping needles only as a last resort.

_____ **27.** A venous access device should be accessed with a(n):
   A. heparin lock.
   B. Huber needle.
   C. over-the-needle catheter.
   D. hollow-needle catheter.

_____ **28.** A Huber needle should be inserted into the injection port at a:
   A. 15-degree angle.
   B. 30-degree angle.
   C. 45-degree angle.
   D. 90-degree angle.

_____ **29.** Complications of using a venous access device include all of the following **except**:
   A. infection.
   B. hypotension.
   C. thrombus formation.
   D. dislodgment of the catheter tip from the vein.

_____ **30.** A complication associated with use of infusion pumps is:
   A. hypotension.
   B. infection.
   C. extravasation.
   D. thrombus formation.

_____ **31.** Situations that may require intraosseous infusion include all of the following **except**:
   A. pneumonia.
   B. shock.
   C. vascular collapse.
   D. trauma.

_____ **32.** Saying "Don't worry, everything will be all right" is an example of:
   A. providing false reassurance.
   B. giving advice.
   C. using avoidance language.
   D. using authority.

_____ **33.** A person who shifts the focus of a conversation rather than getting into a discussion of something difficult is using:
   A. reflective language.
   B. interpretive technique.
   C. avoidance language.
   D. dissemination technique.

_____ **34.** Magical thinking begins at:
   A. 12-18 months.
   B. 18-24 months.
   C. 24-36 months.
   D. 36-48 months.

_____ **35.** A child's hearing reaches maturity at:
   A. 12-18 months.
   B. 2-3 years.
   C. 3-4 years.
   D. 5-6 years.

_____ **36.** When oxygen is combined with hemoglobin, it is measured as:
   A. oxygen saturation.
   B. partial pressure of oxygen.
   C. partial pressure of carbon dioxide.
   D. carbon dioxide saturation.

_____ **37.** When atelectasis is present, which gas exchange is taking place?
   A. Oxygen to carbon dioxide
   B. Carbon dioxide to oxygen
   C. Oxygen to nitrogen
   D. No gas exchange is taking place.

_____ **38.** Which of the following refers to the concentration of oxygen in inspired air?
   A. PaO_2
   B. HCO_3
   C. FiO_2
   D. $PaCO_2$

_____ **39.** Decreased partial pressure of oxygen in the blood is called:
   A. hypoxia.
   B. hypoxic drive.
   C. hypercarbia.
   D. hypoxemia.

_____ **40.** An oxygen deficiency is called:
   A. hypoxia.
   B. hypoxic drive.
   C. hypercarbia.
   D. hypoxemia.

_____ **41.** The automatic transport ventilator is contraindicated for all of the following patients **except** an intubated:
   A. 4-year-old near drowning victim.
   B. 17-year-old gunshot victim.
   C. 34-year-old with adult respiratory distress syndrome.
   D. 56-year-old in pulmonary edema.

_____ **42.** A tank containing liquid oxygen should be stored:
    A. on its side.
    B. upright.
    C. cylinder valve side down.
    D. in any manner that is convenient.

_____ **43.** All of the following are indications of proper endotracheal tube placement **except**:
    A. absence of breath sounds over the epigastrium.
    B. presence of condensation inside the endotracheal tube.
    C. poor compliance with mechanical ventilation.
    D. absence of phonation once the tube is placed.

_____ **44.** When an endotracheal tube is inserted too far, it usually tends to enter the:
    A. trachea.
    B. primary bronchus.
    C. pericardium.
    D. right mainstem bronchus.

_____ **45.** You can provide humidified oxygen to the patient by attaching a reservoir of:
    A. lactated ringers.
    B. non-sterile saline.
    C. sterile-water.
    D. distilled water.

_____ **46.** Part of active listening includes maintaining eye contact and using appropriate gestures in a process known as:
    A. formulation.
    B. facilitation.
    C. fulmination.
    D. facultation.

_____ **47.** A tear in the tracheo-bronchial tree or a pneumothorax can be characterized by _____ in the neck.
    A. subcutaneous emphysema
    B. swollen lymph nodes
    C. mediastinal deviation
    D. jugular venous distention

_____ **48.** _____ respiration is characterized by tachypnea and hyperpnea.
    A. Kussmaul's
    B. Biot's
    C. Cheyne-Stokes
    D. Apneustic

_____ **49.** The standard sequence for examining the chest is:
    A. inspect, palpate, auscultate, percuss.
    B. palpate, percuss, auscultate, inspect.
    C. inspect, auscultate, percuss, palpate.
    D. inspect, palpate, percuss, auscultate.

_____ **50.** When documenting exam findings, a paramedic should record:
  A. only positive findings.
  B. everything.
  C. only negative findings.
  D. his interpretation of patient statements.

_____ **51.** One generally accepted method for organizing patient charts is the _____ format.
  A. ABCDE
  B. PQRST-PLAN
  C. SOAP
  D. ALS-RUN

_____ **52.** School-age children (4-10 years) should:
  A. undergo the same physical exam as an adult.
  B. be allowed to participate in the exam.
  C. have their parents answer all questions.
  D. have invasive procedures performed first.

_____ **53.** Patients with serious illness or injury should be transported immediately:
  A. in order for paramedics to return and treat additional patients.
  B. because a physician is required to perform a complete assessment.
  C. because it reduces the liability of the paramedics.
  D. to get the patient to a facility that can deliver definitive care.

_____ **54.** A patient _____ is an example of one requiring expeditious transport.
  A. with an isolated wrist fracture
  B. with neck and back pain secondary to a motor vehicle collision
  C. who complains of burns from the air bag
  D. who is unresponsive to stimuli

_____ **55.** _____ is (are) a reliable indicator of circulatory/cardiovascular status function in infants and children.
  A. Blood pressure
  B. Capillary refill
  C. Electrocardiogram findings
  D. Skin temperature

_____ **56.** You should conduct a thorough and comprehensive examination of the entire body during the:
  A. initial assessment.
  B. rapid trauma assessment.
  C. detailed physical exam.
  D. ongoing assessment.

_____ **57.** In any significantly traumatized person, what phase of the assessment format is **most** **likely** to be skipped without detriment to the patient?
  A. The scene sizeup
  B. The rapid trauma assessment
  C. The initial assessment
  D. The detailed physical exam

_____ **58.** Which of the following is a mnemonic for the signs to look for during a detailed physical exam?
   A. SAMPLE
   B. DCAP-BTLS
   C. OPQRST
   D. AEIOU

_____ **59.** <u>Scenario</u>: Your 23-year-old female patient presents with relatively normal vital signs and is fully alert and oriented. Her only complaint is lower abdominal pain. If you assume she is pregnant you are:
   A. applying the principles.
   B. evaluating.
   C. overgeneralizing.
   D. interpreting the data.

_____ **60.** During the ongoing assessment of a stable patient, you should recheck vital signs every 15 minutes. This is an example of:
   A. applying the principles.
   B. reflecting.
   C. reviewing.
   D. evaluating.

_____ **61.** _____ communications are condensed and require a decoder to translate.
   A. Analog
   B. Telephone
   C. Cellular
   D. Digital

_____ **62.** Cellular telephone systems use _____ to transmit communications.
   A. regional radio base stations
   B. computers
   C. digital technology
   D. multiple radio frequencies

_____ **63.** A _____ reads printed information and transmits it to another machine.
   A. computer
   B. facsimile machine
   C. trunking machine
   D. touch pad

_____ **64.** The **final** step in the communications process is:
   A. decoding.
   B. feedback.
   C. encoding.
   D. receiving.

_____ **65.** _____ should read and review the PCR before you submit it as complete.
   A. No one but you
   B. No one but you and your partner
   C. No one but you, your partner, and the patient
   D. Everyone involved in the call

_____ **66.** The PCR should be completed immediately after the call because:
   A. the information is fresh in your mind.
   B. the receiving facility demands it.
   C. the medical control physician must sign it.
   D. you need to get back in service.

_____ **67.** The format that uses a <u>chronological</u> <u>account</u> from the time of arrival on scene to the time of transfer of care is known as:
   A. objective-subjective.
   B. SOAP.
   C. call incident.
   D. patient management.

_____ **68.** The call incident approach for narrative writing emphasizes all of the following <u>except</u>:
   A. absolute chronological order.
   B. mechanism of injury.
   C. surrounding circumstances.
   D. how the incident occurred.

_____ **69.** As a bullet tumbles, its potential to inflict damage:
   A. remains the same.
   B. decreases.
   C. increases.
   D. is determined by the trajectory.

_____ **70.** A bullet's characteristics determine how much damage it creates as it strikes its target. Which of the following would create the <u>most</u> damage?
   A. A full-metal-jacket bullet
   B. A small-profile bullet
   C. A bullet that does not tumble
   D. A bullet that flattens when it hits

_____ **71.** The <u>leading</u> cause of death in persons under the age of 44 is:
   A. heart attack.
   B. cancer.
   C. cardiovascular disease.
   D. trauma.

_____ **72.** Some trauma centers commit to special emergency department training and have a degree of surgical capability. This center is designated as:
   A. Level I.
   B. Level II.
   C. Level III.
   D. Level IV.

_____ **73.** Which of the following patients would you expect to show signs of hypovolemic shock?
   A. Pulse of 90 in an adult
   B. Pulse of 140 in an infant
   C. Pulse of 110 in a preschooler
   D. Pulse of 130 in a teenager

_____ **74.** Your patient has been compensating for shock, and his vitals are holding steady. There is a significant mechanism of injury. How should you transport this patient?
  A. No load
  B. Low priority
  C. Rapid transport
  D. Instruct the patient to follow up with his family doctor

_____ **75.** If available, which IV cannulation site would be **best** for the trauma victim in need of extensive fluid resuscitation?
  A. Dorsum of the hand
  B. Forearm
  C. Antecubital fossa
  D. External jugular

_____ **76.** Small capillary injuries like abrasions and paper cuts may continue to ooze and bleed for a short time because:
  A. capillaries are under high pressure.
  B. capillary blood does not contain platelets.
  C. capillaries cannot contract.
  D. capillaries carry large amounts of blood.

_____ **77.** Any injury in which the skin is broken is referred to as:
  A. a fracture.
  B. a musculoskeletal injury.
  C. a closed wound.
  D. an open wound.

_____ **78.** <u>Scenario</u>: You are dispatched to a building collapse with several trapped patients who will require very long extrications. Which of the following medications would you consider giving your patient to combat the effects of acidosis?
  A. Valium
  B. Oxygen
  C. Sodium bicarbonate
  D. Morphine

_____ **79.** Which type of tissue is affected in an airway thermal burn?
  A. Striated muscle
  B. Mucosa
  C. Smooth muscle
  D. Fascia

_____ **80.** The major problem with an airway inhalation burn is:
  A. hypoxia.
  B. shock.
  C. systemic poisoning.
  D. tissue edema.

_____ **81.** Electricity can affect muscle. When electricity affects cardiac muscle, it can cause a deadly rhythm that is called:
  A. wandering pacemaker.
  B. ventricular fibrillation.
  C. supraventricular tachycardia.
  D. bradycardia.

_____ **82.** When a patient comes into contact with a source of electricity, the smaller the area of contact, the _____ the injury.
  A. smaller
  B. more superficial
  C. greater
  D. more obvious

_____ **83.** <u>Scenario</u>: You arrive on scene and find a patient involved in an automobile accident. The patient does not respond to painful stimuli, has a fixed and dilated pupil, with muscle flaccidity on the left. Your **initial** field diagnosis would be:
  A. spinal cord transection.
  B. head injury.
  C. significant hypoxemia.
  D. spinal shock.

_____ **84.** <u>Scenario</u>: After taking the vital signs you find a B/P of 82/60, HR 132, RR 8 and irregular with a capillary refill of 4 seconds. The vitals should cause you to suspect:
  A. hidden hemorrhage elsewhere in the body.
  B. Cushing's reflex.
  C. diffuse axonal injury.
  D. spinal shock.

_____ **85.** Which of the following drugs used in head injury patients would lessen ICP by pulling fluid into the vascular compartment?
  A. Furosemide
  B. Mannitol
  C. Solumedrol
  D. Succinylcholine

_____ **86.** Which of the following drugs is administered to a head-injury patient at a dose of 0.5 to 1.0 mg/kg?
  A. Vecuronium
  B. Succinylcholine
  C. Furosemide
  D. Morphine

_____ **87.** Which of the following involves a bruising of the spinal cord?
  A. Laceration
  B. Concussion
  C. Compression
  D. Contusion

_____ **88.** Which of the following are you **least** **likely** to consider during your scene sizeup?
   A. Mechanism of injury
   B. Falls greater than three times the patient's height
   C. Hemiparesis or paralysis
   D. Identification of likely movements of the spine during the crash or impact

_____ **89.** Scenario: A 30-year-old patient who was involved in a motorcycle accident complains of pain at L-3 that radiates to both legs. Upon palpation of the cervical spine, you note deformity in this same area. After you have completed your scene survey and initial assessment, which of the following would be the logical **next** step in your evaluation process?
   A. Perform a rapid trauma assessment en route to the tertiary care center.
   B. Perform a rapid trauma assessment on scene prior to loading the patient in the ambulance.
   C. Perform a focused history and physical exam prior to transport.
   D. Repeat your initial assessment prior to completing your focused history and physical exam.

_____ **90.** Scenario: You arrive on the scene of an MVA involving a 26-year-old male. The patient presents with a blood pressure of 90 mmHg systolic, weak peripheral pulses, and loss of muscle tone and apnea. Under your suspicion that a spinal cord injury has occurred, where do you suspect nerve transmission has been disrupted?
   A. The phrenic nerve (C1-C3)
   B. The phrenic nerve (C3-C5)
   C. The lumbar plexus (L1-L5)
   D. The brachial plexus (T6-T9)

_____ **91.** Which of the following would you be **least** **likely** to evaluate during scene sizeup?
   A. Mental status
   B. Scene safety
   C. Mechanism of injury
   D. Type and caliber of weapon

_____ **92.** Which of the following statements about percussing the thorax is **correct**?
   A. Hyporesonance indicates excess air in the lungs.
   B. Hyporesonance indicates excess fluid or blood in the lungs.
   C. Hyperresonance indicates excess fluid or blood in the lungs.
   D. Hyperresonance is a normal finding.

_____ **93.** <u>Scenario</u>: You are called to the scene for a two-car MVA. Upon approaching the patient, you note major damage to the front end of the vehicle as well as a bent steering wheel. The patient complains of chest pain and shortness of breath. Your assessment reveals a blood pressure of 90 systolic, weak radial pulses with a rate of 120, and a respiratory rate of 26 and shallow. The cardiac monitor reveals sinus tachycardia with PVCs. Based on the mechanism of injury and the patient's presentation, which of the following injuries might you suspect?
   A. Myocardial aneurysm
   B. Abdominal aortic aneurysm
   C. Pulmonary contusion
   D. Myocardial contusion

_____ **94.** Which of the following is the **<u>most</u> <u>appropriate</u>** management for a patient with a traumatic rupture of the aorta?
   A. Begin a dopamine infusion at 5 mcg/kg/min prior to transport.
   B. Delay transport to apply MAST trousers.
   C. Initiate two large-bore IVs on scene.
   D. Expedite transport to a trauma center for surgical intervention.

_____ **95.** The peritoneum protects the abdominal contents from movement, temperature extremes, and infection. The double fold of peritoneal tissue that suspends the bowel from the posterior abdomen is the:
   A. peritoneal lavage.
   B. lesser omentum.
   C. mesentery.
   D. greater aortic ligament.

_____ **96.** Using a pneumatic antishock garment is a consideration in the hypovolemic patient. Select the correct statement regarding PASG use.
   A. Do not inflate the abdominal compartment of the PASG in an evisceration of the bowel.
   B. The PASG may be used to stabilize an impaled object in the abdomen.
   C. PASG use should be considered only if it is possible to return the patient to his pre-injury state.
   D. Never use the PASG device in a pregnant female patient.

_____ **97.** In addition to applying any immobilization device, it is imperative that pulse, motor functions, and sensation in the extremity distal to the injury site be evaluated. This should be done:
   A. only after the splinting device is fully in place to assure that adjustments do not cause further impairments.
   B. before and after the application of any immobilization device.
   C. only in the conscious, adult patient who is able to understand and follow commands.
   D. just prior to arrival at the ER to assure that your report is accurate and concise.

_____ **98.** Which of the following statements about injuries to the elbow **is** **true**?
  A. They seldom involve nerves and blood vessels and are, therefore, of little risk to the patient.
  B. They have a high probability of involving the brachial nerve and radial artery.
  C. They can be managed by the use of a rigid splint.
  D. They must be managed by keeping the wrist below the level of the elbow to ensure venous return.

_____ **99.** Fractures to the shoulder **most** **commonly** involve the proximal humerus, lateral scapula, and distal scapula. Shoulder injuries **without** **pulse** **deficit** should be managed by:
  A. single reduction attempts followed by sling and swathe.
  B. repeat reduction attempts until deformity is aligned.
  C. immobilization in position found.
  D. aligning the affected limb into the axillary region and securing it to thorax using cravats or 3-inch cling.

_____ **100.** Diazepam, or Valium, is a benzodiazepine with both anxiolytic and skeletal muscle relaxant properties, and can be administered prehospitally for pain management. The **most** **appropriate** dosing regimen for Valium is:
  A. mix prescribed amount of diazepam into 50 ml bag of normal saline and infuse over 10 minutes.
  B. administer 5-15 g diazepam IV push, close to the site of cannulation.
  C. administer 5-15 mg diazepam IV push, close to the site of cannulation.
  D. mix 5 mg diazepam into 2 ml of flumazenil, close to the site of cannulation.

_____ **101.** The respiratory pattern that is characterized by long, deep breaths separated by periods of apnea is known as:
  A. apneustic.
  B. Biot's.
  C. Cheyne-Stokes breathing.
  D. Kussmaul's.

_____ **102.** **Scenario:** A 24-year-old male has been pulled from the water after being submerged for 10 minutes. He is unconscious, unresponsive, apneic, and pulseless. CPR with BVM and supplemental oxygen is being provided to the patient, but the patient still remains cyanotic. The **most** **likely** reason for poor lung diffusion is the:
  A. concentration of oxygen delivered to the alveoli.
  B. interstitial thickness of the alveoli.
  C. perfusion of the alveoli.
  D. patency of the alveoli.

_____ **103.** Pulse oximetry measures the:
  A. arterial blood analysis of oxygen dissolved in plasma.
  B. arterial blood analysis of carbon dioxide dissolved in plasma.
  C. desaturation of hemoglobin with carbon dioxide.
  D. saturation of hemoglobin with oxygen.

_____**104.** Which of the following devices evaluates the patient's expiratory efficiency?
    A. Capnometry
    B. Pulse oximetry
    C. Sphygmomanometer
    D. Spirometer

_____**105.** <u>Scenario</u>: A 42-year-old female awakens suddenly in the middle of the night with severe dyspnea. She gave birth two weeks ago. In addition to her symptoms, you would expect to see all of the following signs <u>except</u>:
    A. labored breathing.
    B. rising blood pressure.
    C. tachypnea.
    D. tachycardia.

_____**106.** <u>Scenario</u>: You encounter a patient with a normal P-R interval, a QRS duration of 0.08, and a R-R interval of 0.48 seconds. This patient is in:
    A. atrial fibrillation.
    B. atrial flutter.
    C. sinus tachycardia.
    D. supraventricular tachycardia.

_____**107.** <u>Scenario</u>: A 16-year-old female is crying and hysterical after breaking up with her boyfriend. She fainted prior to EMS arrival and is presently A&Ox4 with vitals of BP 112/72, P 96 and irregular, and R of 36 crying. After placing her on the cardiac monitor, you note that she has a normal P-R interval, QRS duration, and T waves. It is safe to assume that her ECG is:
    A. sinus arrest.
    B. sinus bradycardia.
    C. sinus dysrhythmia.
    D. sinus tachycardia.

_____**108.** <u>Scenario</u>: A 62-year-old male fainted while going to the bathroom. His current vitals are blood pressure 108/64, pulse 62 and irregular, and respirations 24. His ECG displays an irregular rhythm with normal P-R interval and QRS complex. The **most** <u>likely</u> cause of the patient's syncopal episode is:
    A. AV-node ischemia.
    B. digitalis toxicity.
    C. excessive vagal tone.
    D. fibrotic disease.

_____**109.** <u>Scenario</u>: EMS is called to the scene of an 82-year-old male with a history of cardiac complications. After placing him on the monitor, you note that the rhythm is slightly irregular with normal QRS complexes, but each P wave is different. This rhythm is:
    A. runs of PACs.
    B. sinus arrest.
    C. sinus dysrhythmia.
    D. wandering pacemaker.

_____ **110.** <u>Scenario</u>: A patient with a history of bronchitis and emphysema is suffering from adult respiratory distress syndrome. ECG monitoring shows a tachycardic rhythm of 132 with varying P-R intervals and irregular P waves. The ECG is:

    A. accelerated sinus dysrhythmia.

    B. atrial fibrillation.

    C. atrial flutter.

    D. multifocal atrial tachycardia.

_____ **111.** <u>Scenario</u>: A 62-year-old male fainted while going to the bathroom. His current vitals are blood pressure 98/64, pulse 42 and irregular, and respirations 24. His ECG displays an irregular rhythm with normal P-R interval and QRS complex. Based upon the information presented, the <u>**best**</u> treatment for this patient is:

    A. atropine 0.5 mg.

    B. epinephrine 1:10,000 1 mg.

    C. isuprel 2-10 mcg/min.

    D. transcutaneous pacing.

_____ **112.** <u>Scenario</u>: A 24-year-old female is complaining of chest pain and difficulty breathing. She has been up for three days studying for finals and has been taking ephedrine supplements to help her stay awake and alert. She also admits to drinking 12 Mountain Dew soft drinks in the past day. Vitals are BP 80/40, P 180 and R 42, and she is very pale and lethargic. Placing her on the ECG monitor, you notice a wave preceding the normal QRS complex, but cannot discern P or T waves. The <u>**best**</u> treatment for this patient would include:

    A. adenosine 6 mg rapid IVP.

    B. cardioversion at 100 joules.

    C. vagal maneuvers.

    D. verapamil 2.5 mg slow IVP.

_____ **113.** <u>Scenario</u>: A 52-year-old male patient is experiencing chest pain and shortness of breath. Vitals are blood pressure 108/64, pulse 50 and irregular, and respirations 36. ECG shows an irregular ventricular rhythm and a P-R interval that becomes progressively longer ending in a nonconducted QRS complex. Which of the following regimens is indicated for this patient?

    A. IV, O_2, adenosine 6 mg

    B. IV, O_2, atropine 0.5 mg

    C. IV, O_2, lidocaine 1.5 mg/kg

    D. IV, O_2, verapamil 2.5 mg

_____ **114.** <u>Scenario</u>: A patient is experiencing severe chest pain and is hemodynamically unstable. ECG shows a ventricular rate of 40. P-R interval is 0.24 and is constant for conducted QRS complexes. However, every 4th P wave does not conduct a QRS. Immediate management for this patient should <u>**include**</u>:

    A. adenosine 6 mg.

    B. atropine 1 mg.

    C. lidocaine 1 mg/kg.

    D. transcutaneous pacing.

_____ **115.** <u>Scenario</u>: A patient involved in a motor vehicle accident is semiconscious. Vitals are blood pressure of 102/64, pulse of 120, and respirations of 24. ECG shows a sinus tachycardia with bigeminy. Which of the following treatments is appropriate?
   A. Immediate cardioversion at 100 joules
   B. Immediate defibrillation at 200 joules
   C. Lidocaine 1 mg/kg
   D. Vagal maneuvers

_____ **116.** Management of a patient with a vascular emergency should consist of:
   A. aggressive IV therapy and administration of a beta adrenergic.
   B. general supportive therapy as indicated by signs and symptoms.
   C. IV at KVO, oxygen, and lasix administration.
   D. oxygen and calm transport.

_____ **117.** Leads aVR, aVL, and aVF are considered:
   A. bipolar leads.
   B. precordial leads.
   C. reciprocal leads.
   D. unipolar leads.

_____ **118.** Which of the following is a precordial lead?
   A. Lead I
   B. aVR
   C. rVR
   D. V1

_____ **119.** This lead is determined by placing the positive electrode to the left of the sternum at the fourth intercostal space.
   A. V1
   B. V2
   C. V3
   D. V4

_____ **120.** The chemical neurotransmitter for the sympathetic innervation of the heart is:
   A. acetylcholine.
   B. adrenaline.
   C. epinephrine.
   D. norepinephrine.

_____ **121.** A sudden, temporary loss of consciousness caused by insufficient blood flow to the brain, with near immediate recovery upon becoming supine is:
   A. a cerebral vascular accident.
   B. a seizure.
   C. syncope.
   D. trigeminal palsy.

_____**122.** <u>Scenario</u>: A 21-year-old female suddenly goes unconscious and slumps to the floor during a college exam. She is pale, diaphoretic, and conscious upon arrival of EMS. She is alert and oriented to person, place, time, and event. Vitals are blood pressure of 110/72, pulse of 98, and respirations of 18. She has no major complaints other than being embarrassed. All of the following procedures would be appropriate **except**:

A. blood glucose analysis.

B. cardioversion.

C. evaluate ECG.

D. reassure the patient.

_____**123.** <u>Scenario</u>: A patient is experiencing a severe throbbing in the temples, with accompanying photosensitivity, nausea, vomiting, and diaphoresis. Which type of headache is this considered?

A. Cluster

B. Migraine

C. Organic

D. Tension

_____**124.** The temporary, involuntary twitching of a muscle group commonly witnessed in patients who have multiple sclerosis, Parkinson's, or Alzheimer's is:

A. dystonia.

B. myoclonus.

C. neuropathy.

D. poliomyelitis.

_____**125.** The neural defect that can be characterized by myelomeningocele, meningocele, or occulta is:

A. ALS.

B. muscular dystrophy.

C. myoclonus.

D. spina bifida.

_____**126.** The defect that presents with normal development of the spinal cord, but with the meninges protruding through a spinal opening is:

A. meningocele.

B. myelomeningocele.

C. myoclonus.

D. occulta.

_____**127.** <u>Scenario</u>: A patient is conscious with slurred speech, is slightly irritable, and has cool, clammy skin. Dextrostix shows 54 mg/dL. The treatment for this patient should include all of the following **except**:

A. administration of oral glucose if the patient is able to swallow.

B. consideration of D_{50} if the patient is unable to follow simple commands.

C. assist patient with self administration of insulin.

D. IV of NS.

_____128. Scenario: A patient presents with diaphoresis, tachycardia, seizures, and cool, clammy skin. A dextrostix reveals 10 mg/dL. This patient is experiencing:
A. diabetic coma.
B. diabetic ketoacidosis.
C. hyperglycemia.
D. hypoglycemia.

_____129. Scenario: A patient has fatigue, progressive weakness, vomiting, diarrhea, hypotension, and a decreased appetite. The ECG monitor shows sinus dysrhythmia with frequent PVCs. All of the following are treatments for managing this disorder except:
A. providing aggressive fluid resuscitation.
B. providing supplemental oxygenation.
C. treating underlying cardiovascular disturbances.
D. administering D_{50} if blood glucose level is less than 50 mg/dL.

_____130. Which of the following precautions should be taken when establishing an IV on a patient with Cushing's syndrome?
A. Be cautious when prepping the IV site due to skin fragility.
B. Do not prep the IV site, due to a decreased susceptibility to infection.
C. Secure the IV site with excessive amounts of tape.
D. Vigorously prep the site by scrubbing with betadine and alcohol.

_____131. Antigens that result in an immediate hypersensitivity reaction cause the immediate release of _____ antibodies.
A. IgA
B. IgE
C. IgG
D. IgM

_____132. The most common route of entry of an allergen in an anaphylactic reaction is:
A. absorption.
B. ingestion.
C. inhalation.
D. injection.

_____133. Inflammation of the appendix results in expansion of its internal diameter and thrombosis of its artery. This can result in:
A. atrophy of the appendix.
B. hypertrophy of the appendix.
C. iatrogenic inflammation of the appendix.
D. necrosis of the appendix.

_____134. McBurney's point, a common site of pain from appendicitis, is located:
A. 1-2 inches above the anterior iliac crests inline with the umbilicus.
B. 2 inches above the umbilicus on the midline.
C. 5 inches above the left iliac crest, midaxillary.
D. in the left lower quadrant.

_____**135.** <u>Scenario</u>: Your patient is complaining of severe right upper abdominal pain. Assessment reveals hepatic enlargement, jaundice, and diaphoresis. Prehospital management of this patient should include all of the following **except**:
   A. anti-inflammatory medication administration.
   B. IV therapy.
   C. phenergan.
   D. support of the ABCs.

_____**136.** <u>Scenario</u>: A patient experiences localized abdominal pain in the midepigastric region after eating. The pain tends to subside with milk; however, today she is experiencing nausea and is pale and diaphoretic. The pain has persisted even after drinking milk. The patient admits to smoking and moderate alcohol consumption. Your course of treatment for her should consist of:
   A. administration of phenergan.
   B. IV of NS with 20 ml/kg fluid bolus.
   C. IV sodium bicarbonate.
   D. supportive therapy.

_____**137.** All of the following might be prerenal causes of acute renal failure **except**:
   A. congestive heart failure.
   B. hemorrhage.
   C. hypertension.
   D. sepsis.

_____**138.** Edema in the face, hands, and feet accompanied by a distended abdomen and a decrease in urination is **most** **likely** due to:
   A. acute renal failure.
   B. congestive heart failure.
   C. pulmonary edema.
   D. shock.

_____**139.** All of the following symptoms are typically consistent with urinary tract infections **except**:
   A. difficulty in beginning and continuing to void.
   B. dysuria.
   C. flank pain.
   D. frequent urge to urinate.

_____**140.** <u>Scenario</u>: A patient has been stung by a scorpion and has burning and tingling, emesis/vomiting, muscle twitching, and salivation. You would also expect to see:
   A. abdominal cramping.
   B. fever.
   C. paralysis.
   D. sweating.

_____ **141.** <u>Scenario</u>: A patient is experiencing redness and swelling on the right arm because of multiple fire ant bites. Your assessment reveals profuse urticaria, facial edema, and tachycardia, and the patient is complaining of a very itchy throat. Which of the following should management <u>include</u>?
   A. Atropine 0.5 mg IVP
   B. Epinephrine 1:1000 3 mg SQ
   C. Oxygen by nonrebreather
   D. Rapid sequence intubation

_____ **142.** <u>Scenario</u>: A patient has been bitten by a snake. Bystanders do not know what kind it was but state that it had red, yellow, and black rings and that the red rings were banded on either side by yellow rings. The patient has generalized numbness and weakness in addition to slurred speech. Which of the following signs or symptoms would you also expect?
   A. Respiratory failure
   B. Dry mouth and mucous membranes
   C. Dysuria
   D. Hyperactivity

_____ **143.** All of the following are components of the hemostatic mechanism <u>except</u>:
   A. coagulation.
   B. granulosis.
   C. platelet plugs.
   D. vascular spasms.

_____ **144.** <u>Scenario</u>: You are called to transport a child with a severe fever. Upon your arrival, the family indicates that the 16-year-old has been undergoing chemotherapy for acute myeologenous leukemia and has not eaten in two days. Your assessment reveals a temperature of 104F and very pale skin; the child is extremely weak. Glucometer reading is 102 mg/dL, pulse of 124, blood pressure of 108/72, and respirations of 34. All of the following might be appropriate treatments <u>except</u>:
   A. 25 gm dextrose 50%.
   B. administration of an analgesic.
   C. establishment of an IV of NS.
   D. oxygen by nonrebreather.

_____ **145.** <u>Scenario</u>: You are doing an emergency transfer of a stable multisystem trauma patient from a regional trauma center to the patient's home hospital. A unit of blood was hung prior to transport by the ICU staff. During the transport, the patient suddenly begins complaining of chest pain. Your assessment reveals facial flushing, tachycardia, wheezing, and fever. Treatment should consist of all of the following <u>except</u>:
   A. changing ALL IV tubing and establishing a line of D5W.
   B. considering 25-50 mg diphenhydramine if itching and hives persist.
   C. considering the administration of furosemide to promote diuresis.
   D. stopping the blood transfusion.

_____**146.** _____ pass easily through clothing and the entire body and are stopped only by lead shielding.
   A. Alpha particles
   B. Beta particles
   C. Gamma particles
   D. Neutrons

_____**147.** With a core temperature of 28°C (82.4°F) a patient will display all of the following signs or symptoms __except__:
   A. decline in oxygen consumption and pulse.
   B. decreased muscle rigidity.
   C. loss of consciousness.
   D. marked bradypnea.

_____**148.** According to Dalton's law, as altitude increases, the partial pressure of oxygen:
   A. decreases.
   B. increases.
   C. remains the same until an altitude of 2,438 feet is reached.
   D. remains the same.

_____**149.** Healthcare providers should have a PPD skin test every:
   A. 3 months.
   B. 6 months.
   C. 12 months.
   D. 24 months.

_____**150.** Lyme disease may result in inflammation of _____ Bell's Palsy.
   A. CN-I
   B. CN-V
   C. CN-VII
   D. CN-XII

─────── **Helpful Hint** ───────

Try to determine why you selected the wrong answer. Usually something influenced your selection. Focus on the difference between your wrong answer and the correct answer. Carefully read and study the entire paragraph containing the correct answer. Highlight the answer just as you did for Examination I-1.

Did you score higher than 80 percent on Examination I-2? Circle Yes or No in ink. (We will return to your answer to this question later in SAEP.)

Now that you have finished the feedback step for Examination I-2, it is time to repeat the process by taking another comprehensive examination of the *DOT National Standard Curriculum for the Paramedic*.

Examination I-3, Confirming What You Mastered

During Examination I-3 progress will be made in reinforcing what you have learned and improving your examination-taking skills. This examination contains approximately 40 percent of the examination items you have already answered and several new examination items. Follow the steps carefully to realize the best return on effort.

Step 1—Take Examination I-3. When you have completed Examination I-3, go to Appendix A and compare your answers with the correct answers.

Step 2—Score Examination I-3. How many examination items did you miss? Write the number of missed examination items in the blank in ink _____. Enter the number of examination items you guessed in this blank _____. Enter these numbers in the designated locations on your Personal Progress Plotter.

Step 3—During the feedback step, research the correct answer using Appendix A information for Examination I-3. Highlight the correct answer during your research of the reference materials. Read the entire paragraph containing the correct answer.

Examination I-3

Directions

Remove Examination I-3 from the manual. First, take a careful look at the examination. There should be 200 examination items. Notice that a blank line precedes each examination-item number. This line is provided for you to enter the answer to the examination item. Write the answer in ink. Remember the rule about not changing your answers. Our research shows that changed answers are most often changed to an incorrect answer, and, more often than not, the answer that is chosen first is correct.

If you guess an answer, place an "X" or a check mark by your answer. This step is vitally important to gain and master knowledge. We will explain how we treat the "guessed" items later in SAEP.

Take the examination. Once you complete it, go to Appendix A and score your examination. Once the examination is scored, carefully follow the directions for feedback of the missed and guessed examination items.

_____ **1.** The process by which an agency or association grants recognition to an individual who has met its qualifications is:
  A. certification.
  B. licensure.
  C. registration.
  D. reciprocity.

_____ **2.** In 1988, the National Highway Traffic Safety Administration defined 10 elements necessary to all EMS systems. Which of the items below **is not** one of those elements?
  A. Medical direction
  B. Consumer participation
  C. Evaluation
  D. Regulation and policy

_____ **3.** The appropriate receiving hospital for a patient suffering multi-system trauma would be a:
  A. Level I facility.
  B. Level II facility.
  C. Level III facility.
  D. Level IV facility.

_____ **4.** Which of the following **is not** one of the standard warning signs of cancer?
  A. Change in a mole
  B. Blood in the stools/unusual discharge
  C. Lumps
  D. Weight gain

_____ **5.** Which of the following **is not** a normal part of the fight-or-flight response?
  A. Heart rate increases
  B. Digestion slows
  C. Blood pressure increases
  D. Pupils constrict

_____ **6.** The <u>leading</u> cause of death from unintentional injuries in the United States is:
   A. motor-vehicle collisions.
   B. sports injuries.
   C. assaults.
   D. hunting accidents.

_____ **7.** The <u>most</u> <u>frequent</u> causes of injuries in children younger than 6 years old are:
   A. burns.
   B. MVCs.
   C. bicycle incidents.
   D. falls.

_____ **8.** Items that paramedics can document on patient forms to help implement future injury prevention programs <u>include</u>:
   A. scene conditions at the time of EMS arrival.
   B. risks that EMS personnel had to overcome.
   C. use or non-use of protective devices.
   D. All of the above.

_____ **9.** A written statement of a patient's own preference for future medical care is a(n):
   A. patient narrative.
   B. deposition.
   C. power of attorney.
   D. advance directive.

_____ **10.** <u>Scenario</u>: You are treating a patient for whom you believe you must start an IV of lactated Ringer's. The patient, however, says he is frightened of needles and refuses to give his consent. If you display the IV catheter and begin to bring it toward him, you may be charged with:
   A. abandonment.
   B. battery.
   C. misfeasance.
   D. assault.

_____ **11.** A paramedic may be responsible for the negligence of EMT-Bs and EMT-Is under his supervision under the:
   A. res ipsa loquitur clause.
   B. elastic clause.
   C. ex parte Milligan decision.
   D. borrowed servant doctrine.

_____ **12.** Which of the following <u>is</u> <u>not</u> a valid reason for releasing confidential patient information?
   A. The patient's other medical care providers have a need to know.
   B. A local newspaper cites the First Amendment right of its readers to the information.
   C. A judge signs a court order requesting the information.
   D. A private insurance company needs the information for billing purposes.

_____ **13.** If a paramedic leaves a patient unattended, even for a short time, he or she is exposed to charges of:
   A. misfeasance.
   B. abandonment.
   C. desertion.
   D. nonfeasance

_____ **14.** Straps, jackets, and blankets are all examples of:
   A. personal protective equipment.
   B. BSI gear.
   C. rescue gear.
   D. restraining devices.

_____ **15.** DNR orders, durable powers of attorney, and living wills are forms of:
   A. depositions.
   B. torts.
   C. advance directives.
   D. interrogatories.

_____ **16.** Paramedics may provide circulatory support through IV fluids and CPR and ventilatory support via endotracheal tube to a clinically dead patient who is:
   A. the subject of a criminal investigation.
   B. the defendant in a criminal trial.
   C. an organ donor.
   D. a member of certain religious groups.

_____ **17.** Which of the following is considered to be the body's first line of defense in preventing infection and injury?
   A. Anatomical barriers
   B. Inflammatory response
   C. Immune response
   D. Body substance isolation

_____ **18.** Which of the following statements about immunity and inflammation **is true**?
   A. Inflammation directly targets specific antigens.
   B. Immunity involves one type of a specific antigen.
   C. Inflammation involves lymphocytes only.
   D. Immunity and inflammation are independent functions.

_____ **19.** The immune response ability begins to develop in:
   A. the toddler.
   B. the infant.
   C. the neonate.
   D. utero.

_____ **20.** Mast cells synthesize prostaglandins, which:
   A. cause pain.
   B. cause increased vascular permeability.
   C. suppress histamine release.
   D. do all of the above.

_____ **21.** Which of the following is a generic name?
    A. Ethyl 1-methyl-4-phenylisonipecotate hydrochloride
    B. Meperidine hydrochloride
    C. Demerol hydrochloride
    D. Meperidine hydrochloride, USP

_____ **22.** Special considerations must be given to pregnant, pediatric, and geriatric patients with regard to medication administration because they:
    A. have difficulty in understanding why medications are given.
    B. present difficulties in establishing IV access that may warrant use of alternative routes.
    C. present with variations in metabolic function, fluid distribution, and body compositions.
    D. may need a different dose or medication.

_____ **23.** In an emergency, which of the following rights of medication administration may be omitted?
    A. Right patient
    B. Right route
    C. Right medication
    D. All rights need to be followed at all times.

_____ **24.** A beta-2 specific agent will cause what physiologic response?
    A. Increased heart rate
    B. Bronchoconstriction
    C. Bronchodilation
    D. Constriction of pupils

_____ **25.** Phase 0 of cardiac cyclic activity in the fast potentials represents depolarization, which can best be described as a rapid:
    A. influx of K^+.
    B. efflux of Ca^{++}.
    C. efflux of Na^+.
    D. influx of Na^+.

_____ **26.** The action of antiplatelet medications, such as aspirin, unlike anticoagulants (Heparin) is to:
    A. inhibit thromboxane A_2 (TXA_2) synthesis, while lysing formed clots.
    B. promote TXA_2 synthesis, while inhibiting clot formation.
    C. antagonize effects of vitamin K.
    D. inhibit TXA_2 synthesis, while preventing further clot formation.

_____ **27.** Analogues of ADH are used to treat:
    A. acromegaly.
    B. Graves' disease.
    C. diabetes insipidus and nocturnal enuresis.
    D. Cushing's disease.

_____ **28.** Loop diuretics act at the loop of Henle by blocking sodium reabsorption and are effective agents in CHF management. Which of the following is a loop diuretic?
　　A. Furosemide (Lasix)
　　B. Spironolactone (Aldactone)
　　C. Chlorothiazide (Diuril)
　　D. Digoxin (Lanoxin)

_____ **29.** Scenario: You begin a procainamide drip in accordance with ACLS protocol and note a widening of the QRS complex and a prolongation of the QT interval. Bearing in mind that this medication is a sodium channel blocker, what accounts for this phenomenon?
　　A. The depolarization rate is increased.
　　B. The depolarization rate is decreased.
　　C. The repolarization rate is increased.
　　D. The repolarization rate is decreased.

_____ **30.** One of the first-line agents in the prehospital treatment of acute hypertensive crisis (diastolic B/P >130) is:
　　A. nifedipine (Procardia).
　　B. verapamil (Calan).
　　C. nitroglycerine.
　　D. diltiazem (Cardizem).

_____ **31.** A 58-year-old man, complaining of severe chest pain, presents with multifocal PVCs at 12/min, refractory to lidocaine and initial synchronized cardioversion. Your **next** attempt at capturing the PVCs should be use of:
　　A. procainamide.
　　B. morphine sulfate.
　　C. ipratropium.
　　D. cetirizine.

_____ **32.** Scenario: A physician orders administration of heparin at 1000 units per hour to a patient. You have on hand 25,000 units of heparin in 500 cc of normal saline. You will use a microdrip set to run this IV infusion. What should the infusion rate be?
　　A. 16 gtts/minute
　　B. 18 gtts/minute
　　C. 20 gtts/minute
　　D. 22 gtts/minute

_____ **33.** All of the following are indications for intravenous access **except**:
　　A. allergy testing.
　　B. fluid and blood replacement.
　　C. drug administration.
　　D. obtaining venous blood specimens.

_____ **34.** Microdrip tubing has how many drops per milliliter?
　　A. 20 gtts per ml
　　B. 40 gtts per ml
　　C. 60 gtts per ml
　　D. 80 gtts per ml

_____ **35.** Extravasation of an IV site is indicated by:
   A. edema at the IV site.
   B. redness of the IV site.
   C. warmth of the IV site.
   D. bleeding at the IV site.

_____ **36.** All of the following are potential complications of intraosseous access **except**:
   A. fracture.
   B. penetration of medullery cavity/infiltration.
   C. pulmonary embolism.
   D. EPS.

_____ **37.** The **simplest** form of body substance isolation/protection is:
   A. donning gloves.
   B. washing hands.
   C. wearing a face mask.
   D. using eye protection.

_____ **38.** Administering an oral medication to a patient who cannot support his airway may result in:
   A. poor absorption of the medication.
   B. the need to repeat the dose of medication.
   C. aspiration into the lungs.
   D. harmful substances after the drug is metabolized.

_____ **39.** Which of the following **is not** an advantage of a nebulizer or metered dose inhaler?
   A. Less medication is needed because it reaches its exact site of action.
   B. Implementing or discontinuing drug delivery is easy.
   C. It is a less expensive method of drug delivery for an EMS system.
   D. Supplemental oxygen administered simultaneously can assist a hypoxic patient.

_____ **40.** Administration of rectal medication too high in the rectum **may** result in:
   A. rectal bleeding.
   B. vomiting and diarrhea.
   C. giving twice the normal dosage of medication.
   D. absorption of the medication into portal circulation.

_____ **41.** An intramuscular injection is given at a:
   A. 15-degree angle.
   B. 45-degree angle.
   C. 90-degree angle.
   D. 100-degree angle.

_____ **42.** Which of the following is the correct sequence for the colored tubes used when drawing blood?
   A. Blue, green, purple, red, gray
   B. Red, blue, green, purple, gray
   C. Purple, green, blue, gray, red
   D. Gray, purple, green, blue, red

_____ **43.** The exchange of common symbols is:
  A. speaking.
  B. listening.
  C. communication.
  D. understanding.

_____ **44.** Using why questions is poor interviewing technique because it:
  A. uses closed-ended questioning.
  B. appears to place blame on the patient.
  C. confuses an elderly patient.
  D. uses leading questioning.

_____ **45.** Echoing a patient's message back to him using your own words is an example of:
  A. facilitation.
  B. clarification.
  C. reflection.
  D. explanation.

_____ **46.** All of the following are pairs of sinuses **except** the:
  A. oropharyngeal sinuses.
  B. ethmoid sinuses.
  C. frontal sinuses.
  D. sphenoid sinuses.

_____ **47.** The hypoxic drive is regulated by:
  A. PaO_2 levels.
  B. $PaCO_2$ levels.
  C. high oxygen saturation percentage.
  D. low oxygen saturation percentage.

_____ **48.** The airflow during a **maximum** exhalation is the:
  A. peak expiratory flow.
  B. tidal volume.
  C. tidal reserve.
  D. functional residual capacity.

_____ **49.** **Most** oxygen and carbon dioxide gas exchange takes place in the:
  A. alveolar ducts.
  B. alveolar sacs.
  C. right mainstem bronchus.
  D. left mainstem bronchus.

_____ **50.** Field extubation can be performed if the patient:
  A. is under the influence of sedatives.
  B. bites the endotracheal tube during unconsciousness.
  C. is awake and able to maintain his own airway.
  D. becomes combative and starts to pull out the tube.

_____ **51.** The lungs receive most of their blood supply from:
   A. pulmonary arteries.
   B. pulmonary veins.
   C. bronchial arteries.
   D. bronchial veins.

_____ **52.** When oxygen is combined with hemoglobin, it is measured as:
   A. oxygen saturation.
   B. partial pressure of oxygen.
   C. partial pressure of carbon dioxide.
   D. carbon dioxide saturation.

_____ **53.** The normal respiratory rate for an infant is:
   A. 20-40 breaths per minute.
   B. 40-60 breaths per minute.
   C. 60-80 breaths per minute.
   D. 80-100 breaths per minute.

_____ **54.** Applying pressure on the cricoid cartilage to ease endotracheal intubation
   is called:
   A. the modified jaw-thrust maneuver.
   B. the head-tilt/chin lift maneuver.
   C. the Heimlich maneuver.
   D. Sellick's maneuver.

_____ **55.** Which oxygen delivery device delivers the <u>highest</u> concentration of oxygen?
   A. Nasal cannula
   B. Venturi mask
   C. Partial rebreather mask
   D. Nonrebreather mask

_____ **56.** Cricoid pressure must be maintained until the intubation is complete to avoid:
   A. hypoxia.
   B. regurgitation.
   C. mucous plus aspiration.
   D. bleeding.

_____ **57.** The proper order to perform rapid sequence intubation on the patient who
   is alert is:
   A. prepare equipment, administer sedative, administer neuromuscular blocker,
      apply Sellick's maneuver.
   B. prepare equipment, administer sedative, apply Sellick's maneuver, administer
      neuromuscular blocker.
   C. administer sedative, apply Sellick's maneuver, prepare equipment, administer
      neuromuscular blocker.
   D. administer sedative, prepare equipment, apply Sellick's maneuver, administer
      neuromuscular blocker.

_____ **58.** To perform a needle cricothyrotomy in a patient who **does** **not** have a suspected cervical spine injury, the patient should be placed:
   A. supine with head and neck hyperextended.
   B. supine with head and neck in neutral position.
   C. in the lateral recumbent position with head and neck hyperextended.
   D. in the lateral recumbent position with head and neck in neutral position.

_____ **59.** Questions that allow the patient to explain a complaint in detail are known as _____ questions.
   A. explicit
   B. personal
   C. closed-ended
   D. open-ended

_____ **60.** A sign or symptom that causes a patient or bystander to request medical help is known as the:
   A. primary problem.
   B. associated symptom.
   C. chief complaint.
   D. present illness.

_____ **61.** Shining a light onto the iris from the lateral side could cause a shadow on the medial side if the patient were suffering from:
   A. glaucoma.
   B. opiate overdose.
   C. conjunctivitis.
   D. hemianopsia.

_____ **62.** Inspection of the maxillary sinuses is accomplished by:
   A. using an otoscope for visualization.
   B. palpating the nose and septum.
   C. palpating under the zygomatic arches.
   D. obstructing one side and watching the patient breathe.

_____ **63.** _____ respiration is characterized by tachypnea and hyperpnea.
   A. Kussmaul's
   B. Biot's
   C. Cheyne-Stokes
   D. Apneustic

_____ **64.** The standard sequence for examining the chest is:
   A. inspect, palpate, auscultate, percuss.
   B. palpate, percuss, auscultate, inspect.
   C. inspect, auscultate, percuss, palpate.
   D. inspect, palpate, percuss, auscultate.

_____ **65.** A condition that makes posterior chest and lung examination difficult is thoracic:
   A. kyphoscoliosis.
   B. asymmetry.
   C. hyperresonance.
   D. egophony.

_____ **66.** When percussing the chest, the finger should lie _____ to and _____ the ribs.
   A. perpendicular, between
   B. parallel, between
   C. perpendicular, across
   D. parallel, over

_____ **67.** Dullness in the chest during percussion of the 3rd to 5th intercostal spaces can be attributed to the:
   A. stomach.
   B. heart.
   C. thyroid gland.
   D. liver.

_____ **68.** Palpation and inspection of the PMI (apical impulse) can reveal certain conditions such as:
   A. enlarged right ventricle.
   B. tension pneumothorax.
   C. cardiac tamponade.
   D. coronary insufficiency.

_____ **69.** The goal of the initial assessment, when dealing with a trauma patient, is to:
   A. identify life threats.
   B. identify and treat life threats.
   C. identify all injuries sustained by the patient.
   D. identify all patients on scene who need to be transported.

_____ **70.** The **best** method for determining responsiveness to painful stimuli or tactile stimulation in an infant patient is to:
   A. flick the soles of her feet.
   B. rub her sternum.
   C. pinch her fingernails.
   D. pinch her cheeks.

_____ **71.** When assessing the chest, any open wounds that are located should be:
   A. covered with a gauze bandage.
   B. sealed with an occlusive dressing.
   C. probed for depth.
   D. drained using a catheter.

_____ **72.** Determining the patient's mental status early in the assessment phase will accomplish all of the following **except**:
   A. allowing the care provider to receive consent to treat if the patient is responsive.
   B. providing a clue of the patient's basic level of oxygenation and perfusion.
   C. establishing a baseline from which future trends in mental status can be made.
   D. enabling the responder to refuse to provide care if none is needed.

_____ **73.** You should conduct a thorough and comprehensive examination of the entire body during the:
  A. initial assessment.
  B. rapid trauma assessment.
  C. detailed physical exam.
  D. ongoing assessment.

_____ **74.** The evolution of the questions asked of a patient after the first question should be driven by:
  A. mechanism of injury.
  B. intensity of pain.
  C. length of illness.
  D. patient's chief complaint.

_____ **75.** The portion of critical thinking dedicated to assessing initial response to treatment and locating less-than-obvious problems is:
  A. revising.
  B. reacting.
  C. reviewing.
  D. reevaluating.

_____ **76.** You arrive on location and begin to read the scene. You do this by:
  A. addressing life threats.
  B. conducting a focused exam.
  C. observing the immediate surroundings.
  D. auscultating the patient's lungs.

_____ **77.** The acronym PSAP stands for:
  A. prehospital safety and prevention.
  B. public safety answering point.
  C. public safety agency paramedics.
  D. paramedic standard answering point.

_____ **78.** A _____ is a computer on which data is entered by touching areas of the display screen.
  A. screen saver
  B. laptop
  C. notebook
  D. touch pad

_____ **79.** A _____ reads printed information and transmits it to another machine.
  A. computer
  B. facsimile machine
  C. trunking machine
  D. touch pad

_____ **80.** The emergency medical dispatcher has just finished interrogating a caller. The **next** step would be for her to:
  A. send a first responder engine company and paramedics.
  B. call the patient's insurance company for preapproval.
  C. send police, fire, and EMS agencies to the call.
  D. follow established guidelines to determine the appropriate level of response.

_____ **81.** The _____ narrative approach **usually** focuses only on the system(s) involved in the current illness or injury.
   A. head-to-toe
   B. body systems
   C. toe-to-head
   D. focused exam

_____ **82.** The PCR should be completed immediately after the call because:
   A. the information is fresh in your mind.
   B. the receiving facility demands it.
   C. the medical control physician must sign it.
   D. you need to get back in service.

_____ **83.** Each vehicle collision progresses through a series of five events, the **last** of which is:
   A. additional impacts.
   B. secondary collisions.
   C. body collision.
   D. organ collision.

_____ **84.** Which of the following statements regarding the differences between adults and children in pedestrian accidents **is true**?
   A. Adults tend to turn toward the vehicle.
   B. Children tend to turn toward the vehicle.
   C. Adults tend to be thrown under the vehicle.
   D. Children tend to be thrown onto the hood of the vehicle.

_____ **85.** The injuries associated with assault rifles are the same as hunting rifles with the difference being:
   A. multiple wounds are more common with assault rifles.
   B. exit wounds are larger.
   C. entrance wounds are smaller.
   D. energy delivery from military ammunition is more severe.

_____ **86.** The mechanism of injury that suggests transport to a trauma center is:
   A. ejection from a vehicle.
   B. a fall from a distance twice the patient's height.
   C. extrication time of less than 20 minutes.
   D. impact speed of 35 mph.

_____ **87.** Normal expiration can **best** be characterized as a(n) _____ process.
   A. passive
   B. active
   C. alternating
   D. somatic

_____ **88.** The transition between normal function and death is called:
   A. homeostasis.
   B. hemorrhage.
   C. exsanguination.
   D. shock.

_____ **89.** The body's response to local hemorrhage is clotting, a three-phase process. In which phase does the smooth muscle contract, reducing the lumen and strength of blood flow through the vessel?

    A. Vascular phase

    B. Aggregate phase

    C. Platelet phase

    D. Coagulation phase

_____ **90.** <u>Scenario</u>: You are dispatched to a patient with a possible allergic reaction. Upon arrival you have a 14-year-old male who has been stung by numerous bees. He looks very anxious and pale and has a pulse of 140, respirations of 24, and a blood pressure of 110/70. The patient tells you he is allergic to bees and has a medication for them at home. From your training, you expect a dump of histamine by the body, which will cause a drop in the patient's blood pressure and result in shock. This is a form of:

    A. distributive shock.

    B. cardiogenic shock.

    C. hypovolemic shock.

    D. obstructive shock.

_____ **91.** Which of the following is the **<u>best</u>** procedure for administering intravenous fluids for shock trauma resuscitation?

    A. One IV with a 16-gauge needle attached to a macrodrip administration set and a 1000 ml bag of NaCl

    B. One IV with an 18-gauge needle attached to blood tubing and a 1000 ml bag of Ringer's

    C. 14- or 16-gauge needles attached to macrodrip administration sets and 1000 ml bags of NaCl or Ringer's

    D. Two IVs with 18-gauge needles attached to blood tubing and 1000 ml bags of Ringer's lactate

_____ **92.** Dynamic skin tension lines are located at the:

    A. knee.

    B. anterior abdomen.

    C. scalp.

    D. anterior chest.

_____ **93.** In which type of soft tissue injury is the skin cut or torn but not completely torn loose from the body?

    A. Avulsion

    B. Abrasion

    C. Amputation

    D. Laceration

_____ **94.** When skeletal muscle is crushed, the tissue undergoes a degenerative process that releases metabolic byproducts, including many toxins. This process is known as traumatic:

    A. rouleaux.

    B. necrosis.

    C. ischemia.

    D. rhabdomyolysis.

_____ **95.** The patient that has been involved in a crush injury needs to be transported rapidly to the hospital due to:
 A. respiratory compromise.
 B. toxins released into the central circulation.
 C. multiple fractures.
 D. cardiogenic shock.

_____ **96.** In some patients, wounds may continue to ooze fluid because of delayed healing due to underlying medical problems. Prehospital management of these wounds **includes**:
 A. frequent dressing changes.
 B. removal of necrotic tissue.
 C. application of topical medications.
 D. infusion of crystalloid solutions.

_____ **97.** <u>Scenario</u>: You are checking a wound that is 2 to 3 days old. The area of the wound is warm and shows signs of lymphangitis. This finding is indicative of:
 A. collagen synthesis.
 B. infection.
 C. neovascularization.
 D. normal healing.

_____ **98.** Blunt trauma can create internal injuries due to the movement of organs inside the body cavities. Which organ(s) can be lacerated by the ligamentum teres?
 A. The liver
 B. The heart
 C. The lungs
 D. The bladder

_____ **99.** <u>Scenario</u>: You respond to a call of an explosion at a local chemical company. On your arrival, the company hazmat team is in action decontaminating patients before they bring them to you. They bring you a 35-year-old male who is experiencing slight respiratory distress. The care that you should provide **first** for this patient is:
 A. an immediate head-to-toe trauma assessment.
 B. high-flow oxygen.
 C. transport to the local trauma center.
 D. auscultating lung sounds.

_____ **100.** Which of the following burns would be classified as a moderate burn?
 A. Full thickness burns less than 2 percent body surface area
 B. Partial thickness burns greater than 30 percent body surface area
 C. Superficial burns less than 50 percent body surface area
 D. Partial thickness burns less than 25 percent body surface area

_____ **101.** When the skin is burned, the cell membrane ruptures, blood coagulates, and structural proteins denature. This area is the zone of:
 A. coagulation.
 B. stasis.
 C. hyperemia.
 D. fluid shift.

_____**102.** Next to the area where the proteins denature is an inflamed area where blood flow is decreased. This is the:

    A. fluid shift zone.

    B. zone of coagulation.

    C. zone of stasis.

    D. zone of hyperemia.

_____**103.** <u>Scenario</u>: You have been dispatched to a call of a burn patient. Upon arrival you have a 23-year-old female who was sunbathing and fell asleep. She is alert and oriented, in moderate pain, and has blisters covering all four extremities. She also has blisters on her abdomen, face, and chest. You should consider this patient to have _____ burns.

    A. superficial

    B. critical

    C. moderate

    D. minor

_____**104.** Electricity can affect muscle. When electricity affects cardiac muscle, it can cause a deadly rhythm that is called:

    A. wandering pacemaker.

    B. ventricular fibrillation.

    C. supraventricular tachycardia.

    D. bradycardia.

_____**105.** Dislodged teeth are best cared for in the prehospital environment by:

    A. placing them in warm milk for transport.

    B. rinsing them with saline and wrapping them in a saline-soaked gauze pad.

    C. rinsing them with saline and placing them in a carbonated cola drink.

    D. rinsing them and placing them in a plastic bag for transport.

_____**106.** All of the following structures serve some type of protective function for the brain <u>except</u>:

    A. the dura mater.

    B. the scalp.

    C. the cerebrospinal fluid.

    D. the cerebrum.

_____**107.** Limitations to the accuracy of the halo-test can include the presence of all of the following <u>except</u>:

    A. nasal fluids.

    B. lacrimal fluids.

    C. blood.

    D. saliva.

_____**108.** <u>Scenario</u>: After taking the vital signs you find a B/P of 82/60, HR 132, RR 8 and irregular with a capillary refill of 4 seconds. The vitals should cause you to suspect:

    A. hidden hemorrhage elsewhere in the body.

    B. Cushing's reflex.

    C. diffuse axonal injury.

    D. spinal shock.

_____**109.** When should high flow oxygen be provided to a significant head trauma patient with diminished orientation?
A. If there is concurrent airway compromise
B. If the patient is to be ventilated mechanically
C. If the patient is not breathing adequately
D. At all times, regardless of method of delivery

_____ **110.** Axons, which serve as extensions of neurons that transmit signals to and from the brain, are found predominately in:
A. white matter.
B. gray matter.
C. posterior medial sulcus.
D. blue matter.

_____ **111.** Which of the following vital signs indicate a potential spinal cord injury?
A. Hypotension, tachycardia, and deep respirations
B. Hypotension, bradycardia, and shallow respirations
C. Hypertension, bradycardia, and shallow respirations
D. Hypertension, tachycardia, and deep respirations

_____ **112.** Which of the following **does** **not** warrant helmet removal?
A. The helmet prevents airway care.
B. The patient complains of excessive sweating beneath the helmet.
C. The helmet prevents the assessment of anticipated injuries.
D. You anticipate an airway or breathing problem.

_____ **113.** Scenario: You arrive on the scene of an MVA involving a 26-year-old male. The patient presents with a blood pressure of 90 mmHg systolic, weak peripheral pulses, loss of muscle tone, and apnea. Under your suspicion that a spinal cord injury has occurred, where do you suspect nerve transmission has been disrupted?
A. The phrenic nerve (C1-C3)
B. The phrenic nerve (C3-C5)
C. The lumbar plexus (L1-L5)
D. The brachial plexus (T6-T9)

_____ **114.** Scenario: You encounter a patient with a suspected spinal cord injury. Which part of your patient assessment should include manual spinal immobilization followed by mechanical immobilization?
A. Scene sizeup
B. Initial assessment
C. Rapid trauma assessment
D. Focused history and physical exam

_____ **115.** In automobile collisions, the type of impact **most** **commonly** associated with aortic rupture is:
A. lateral.
B. frontal.
C. rollover.
D. rotational.

_____ **116.** Central chemoreceptors respond to changes in:
  A. carbon dioxide and pH in the cerebrospinal fluid.
  B. hydrogen ion concentration in the cerebrospinal fluid.
  C. oxygen and pH in the cerebrospinal fluid.
  D. bicarbonate and hydrogen ion concentration in the cerebrospinal fluid.

_____ **117.** Which of the following would cause a low-energy penetrating wound?
  A. Military M-16 rifle
  B. 12-gauge shotgun
  C. Hunting knife
  D. AK-47 automatic rifle

_____ **118.** Which of the following **most accurately** depicts the chest wall movement in a patient with a flail segment?
  A. Inward with inspiration and outward with expiration
  B. Inward with expiration and outward with inspiration
  C. Inward with both inspiration and expiration
  D. Outward with both inspiration and expiration

_____ **119.** A late sign in a patient with a massive hemothorax would be:
  A. hypertension.
  B. tachycardia.
  C. flat neck veins.
  D. respiratory difficulty/dyspnea.

_____ **120.** Which of the following **best** describes the effects of a pericardial tamponade on cardiac output and venous pressure?
  A. Cardiac output is low, and central venous pressure rises.
  B. Cardiac output is high, and central venous pressure falls.
  C. Cardiac output is not affected, and central venous pressure rises.
  D. Cardiac output rises, and venous pressure is not affected.

_____ **121.** <u>Scenario</u>: You have encountered a patient with a suspected myocardial contusion. In light of the heart's location in their thorax, the chambers that would **most likely** be injured are:
  A. the right and left atria.
  B. the right atrium and right ventricle.
  C. the right and left ventricles.
  D. the left atrium and left ventricle.

_____ **122.** All of the following are functions of the liver **except**:
  A. detoxification of blood.
  B. erythrocytic removal.
  C. cellular glucose metabolism.
  D. osmotic regulation.

_____ **123.** Functions of the pancreas **include**:
  A. destroying aged RBCs.
  B. producing new RBCs.
  C. secreting glucagon.
  D. producing new WBCs.

_____**124.** When hollow organs are injured they can spill their contents causing further damage to the surrounding tissue. Which of the following sets includes **only** hollow organs?
A. Stomach, liver, urinary bladder, esophagus
B. Liver, urinary bladder, kidney, colon
C. Bladder, stomach, colon, esophagus
D. Kidneys, esophagus, gall bladder, spleen

_____**125.** The musculoskeletal system is a complex arrangement of levers and fulcrums providing motion and support for the body. All of the following are functions of the musculoskeletal system **except**:
A. glycogen storage.
B. protection of vital organs.
C. production of blood cells.
D. essential salt storage.

_____**126.** Bone is a living structure that has cells involved in numerous functions of repair and propagation. Identify the function associated with osteoblasts.
A. Maintenance of essential salts and collagen
B. Laying down of new bone in areas of growth and injury
C. Dissolving of bone structure when essential salt demand is high
D. Production of stem cells in red blood cell synthesis

_____**127.** In addition to applying any immobilization device, it is imperative that pulse, motor functions, and sensation in the extremity distal to the injury site be evaluated. This should be done:
A. only after the splinting device is fully in place to assure that adjustments do not cause further impairments.
B. before and after the application of any immobilization device.
C. only in the conscious, adult patient who is able to understand and follow commands.
D. just prior to arrival at the ER to assure that your report is accurate and concise.

_____**128.** Average tidal volume in an adult male is **approximately**:
A. 500 ml.
B. 1200 ml.
C. 3000 ml.
D. 3600 ml.

_____**129.** Chemoreceptors monitor changes in:
A. arterial PCO_2.
B. arterial PO_2.
C. venous PCO_2.
D. venous PO_2.

_____**130.** A dull sound when percussing the chest indicates:
A. ascites.
B. emphysema.
C. pneumothorax.
D. pulmonary edema.

_____ **131.** Pulse oximetry measures the:
  A. arterial blood analysis of oxygen dissolved in plasma.
  B. arterial blood analysis of carbon dioxide dissolved in plasma.
  C. desaturation of hemoglobin with carbon dioxide.
  D. saturation of hemoglobin with oxygen.

_____ **132.** All of the following are characteristic of the second phase reaction of an asthma attack <u>except</u>:
  A. decreased expiratory air flow.
  B. inflammation of the bronchioles.
  C. loss of surfactant in the alveoli.
  D. swelling of the bronchioles.

_____ **133.** If inhaled, which of the following could result in the formation for corrosive acids or alkalis in the airway?
  A. Ammonium hydroxide
  B. Carbon monoxide
  C. Dihydrogen oxide
  D. Nitrous oxide

_____ **134.** The interval from the end of one cardiac contraction to the end of the next is known as:
  A. the cardiac cycle.
  B. diastole.
  C. the heart beat.
  D. systole.

_____ **135.** The intrinsic rate of the _____ is 40-60 beats per minute.
  A. AV node
  B. bundle of His
  C. Purkinje system
  D. SA node

_____ **136.** Changes in the S-T segment might indicate any of the following <u>except</u>:
  A. ischemia.
  B. injury.
  C. infarct.
  D. inotropy.

_____ **137.** When the ECG paper is traveling at 25 mm/sec, an upward deflection on the vertical axis of 2 large boxes indicates a:
  A. negative deflection of 2.0 mV.
  B. negative deflection of 1.0 mV.
  C. positive deflection of 2.0 mV.
  D. positive deflection of 1.0 mV.

_____ **138.** All of the following are typical causes of cardiac dysrhythmia <u>except</u>:
  A. atelectasis.
  B. hypothermia.
  C. myocardial ischemia.
  D. metabolic acidosis.

_____**139.** Which of the following **is not** recommended to use when evaluating an ECG strip?
   A. Analysis of the rate
   B. Analysis of the P waves
   C. Analysis of the QRS complex
   D. Analysis of the T wave

_____**140.** Scenario: A 16-year-old female is crying and hysterical after breaking up with her boyfriend. She fainted prior to EMS arrival and is presently A&Ox4 with vitals of BP 112/72, P 96 and irregular, and R of 36 crying. After placing her on the cardiac monitor, you note that she has a normal P-R interval, QRS duration, and T waves. It is safe to assume that her ECG is:
   A. sinus arrest.
   B. sinus bradycardia.
   C. sinus dysrhythmia.
   D. sinus tachycardia.

_____**141.** Scenario: Your patient is complaining of shortness of breath with a respiratory rate of 36. After applying oxygen via nonrebreather, you place the ECG. Lead II shows P-P intervals of 0.20 seconds and R-R intervals of 0.80 seconds. The rhythm is regular and conduction appears to be 4:1. This ECG indicates:
   A. atrial fibrillation.
   B. atrial flutter.
   C. sinus dysrhythmia.
   D. wandering pacemaker.

_____**142.** A junctional tachycardia rhythm with a rate of 150 may be identified as:
   A. atrial flutter.
   B. sinus tachycardia.
   C. supraventricular tachycardia.
   D. ventricular tachycardia.

_____**143.** Which of the following rules is appropriate for determining a ventricular escape rhythm?
   A. Pacemaker site at the SA node
   B. P waves inverted
   C. Rate greater than 60
   D. QRS duration greater than 0.12

_____**144.** Scenario: A patient has a complete AV dissociation, occasional beats that appear without a P wave, and a QRS complex of 0.24. The ectopic beat is a:
   A. PAC.
   B. PJC.
   C. PVC.
   D. junctional ectopic beat.

_____**145.** Which of the following **is not** an assessment priority when evaluating a patient suspected of suffering an AMI?
   A. Blood pressure
   B. Breath sounds
   C. ECG
   D. Pupilary response

_____**146.** Your patient has had steadily worsening chest pain for 4 hours. He has not had relief with Nitrostat. **Most** **likely** this patient is experiencing:
  A. myocardial infarction.
  B. Prinzmetal's angina.
  C. stable angina.
  D. vasospastic angina.

_____**147.** Which of the following medications and dosages **is** **correct** for the CHF patient?
  A. Furosemide 10 mg
  B. Intropin 5 to 15 mcg/kg/min
  C. Morphine sulfate 20 mg
  D. Promethazine 50 mg

_____**148.** Pulsus alternans occurs when a pulse alternates between:
  A. slow and fast.
  B. normal and inverted.
  C. weak and strong.
  D. regular and irregular.

_____**149.** The body attempts to compensate for cardiogenic shock by:
  A. decreasing chronotropic effects.
  B. decreasing inotropic effects.
  C. increasing contractile force.
  D. increasing peripheral vascular resistance.

_____**150.** An early sign of cardiogenic shock may present as:
  A. altered mental status.
  B. decreased peripheral pulses.
  C. restlessness.
  D. systolic pressure less than 80 mmhg.

_____**151.** Which of the following statements regarding termination of resuscitation efforts in the field **is** **not** true?
  A. EMS personnel should consult with medical control regarding termination efforts.
  B. EMS should notify law enforcement.
  C. The paramedic should discard the ECG tracings, since the patient was not resuscitated.
  D. The paramedic should document all therapy performed.

_____**152.** Unequal bilateral blood pressures in the arms may indicate:
  A. an abdominal aortic aneurysm.
  B. a high thoracic aneurysm.
  C. a cerebral aneurysm.
  D. a subclavian aneurysm.

_____**153.** The number of vertebrae comprising the thoracic spine is:
  A. 4.
  B. 5.
  C. 7.
  D. 12.

_____**154.** The region of the brain that controls eye movement is the:
  A. diencephalon.
  B. encephalon.
  C. mesenchephalon.
  D. triencephalon.

_____**155.** <u>Scenario</u>: A 23-year-old athlete collapses on the track while warming up for track practice. The trainers call EMS. Upon arrival you are informed that the patient experienced generalized muscular spasms for approximately one minute. During your evaluation of the patient, he experiences localized muscle spasms in his right leg that rapidly progress to the entire body. The patient is cyanotic with hypertonic neck muscles noted. Which of the following is an appropriate management?
  A. Administration of 5 mg morphine sulfate
  B. Aggressive management of the airway
  C. Placing a bite stick between the teeth
  D. Restraining the patient

_____**156.** <u>Scenario</u>: A 21-year-old female suddenly goes unconscious and slumps to the floor during a college exam. She is pale, diaphoretic, and conscious upon arrival of EMS. She is alert and oriented to person, place, time, and event. Vitals are blood pressure of 110/72, pulse of 98, and respirations of 18. She has no major complaints other than being embarrassed. All of the following procedures would be appropriate **except**:
  A. blood glucose analysis.
  B. cardioversion.
  C. evaluate ECG.
  D. reassure the patient.

_____**157.** The cause for **most** neoplasms is:
  A. elevated cholesterol.
  B. genetic.
  C. linked to birth control.
  D. relatively unknown.

_____**158.** An abnormal formation in the brain that forms **after** birth is known as a:
  A. congenital neoplasm.
  B. meningocele.
  C. neoplasm.
  D. occulta.

_____**159.** Tissue plasminogen activator administration should begin in the stroke patient within:
  A. 1 hour.
  B. 3 hours.
  C. 6 hours.
  D. 12 hours.

_____**160.** A group of genetic diseases that are characterized by progressive muscle weakness and degeneration of the skeletal, or voluntary, muscles is:
A. Bell's palsy.
B. muscular dystrophy.
C. multiple sclerosis.
D. Parkinson's disease.

_____**161.** Which hormone causes uterine contraction and lactation?
A. Antidiuretic hormone
B. Calcitonin
C. Follicle-stimulating hormone
D. Oxytocin

_____**162.** In the initial phase of diabetic ketoacidosis, profound hyperglycemia exists due to lack of insulin. Consequently, the cells are unable to take in glucose. The compensatory mechanism for this is:
A. glucolysis.
B. gluconeogenesis.
C. glycolysis.
D. glyconeogenesis.

_____**163.** The onset of diabetic ketoacidosis is within:
A. 1-2 hours.
B. 4-8 hours.
C. 6-12 hours.
D. 48 hours.

_____**164.** Scenario: A patient presents with sweet, fruity breath odor, Kussmaul's respirations, and a dextrostix of 268 mg/dL. You should perform all of the following therapies **except**:
A. administering dextrose 50%.
B. establishing an IV of NS.
C. providing oxygen via nonrebreather.
D. collecting a red-top tube of blood.

_____**165.** Scenario: A patient presents with excessive diuresis, dehydration, and a blood glucose of 958, but no ketone breath odor. The absence of ketoacidosis is probably due to:
A. depressed insulin levels.
B. gluconeogenesis.
C. glycolysis.
D. normal insulin level.

_____**166.** Scenario: A patient with hyperglycemic hyperosmolar nonketotic coma is experiencing signs and symptoms of dry skin, flu-like symptoms persisting over several days, tachycardia, and polydipsia. Which of the following signs and symptoms would you also expect to find?
A. Cool skin
B. Kussmaul's respirations
C. Orthostatic hypotension
D. Sweet, fruity breath odor

_____**167.** All of the following are signs or symptoms of myxedema **except**:
    A. cold intolerance.
    B. decreased appetite with increased weight.
    C. decreased mental function.
    D. hyperactivity.

_____**168.** Scenario: A 62-year-old patient is in respiratory failure. Assessment reveals that he has very thin hair, his skin is cool, his tongue is enlarged, and his skin is doughy and edematous. Management should consist of:
    A. infusing warm IV fluids and warm, humidified oxygen.
    B. placing hot packs in his groin and armpits and around his neck.
    C. providing supportive management including intubation and ventilatory assistance.
    D. wrapping him with hot blankets.

_____**169.** Scenario: A patient has fatigue, progressive weakness, vomiting, diarrhea, hypotension, and a decreased appetite. The ECG monitor shows sinus dysrhythmia with frequent PVCs. All of the following are treatments for managing this disorder **except**:
    A. providing aggressive fluid resuscitation.
    B. providing supplemental oxygenation.
    C. treating underlying cardiovascular disturbances.
    D. administering D_{50} if blood glucose level is less than 50 mg/dL.

_____**170.** Scenario: Shortly after being stung by a bee, a patient is experiencing urticaria, stridor, and abdominal cramping. Which of the following signs or symptoms would probably also be present?
    A. Bradycardia
    B. Hypertension
    C. Rhonchi
    D. Wheezing

_____**171.** Which of the following medications is an antiemetic used to comfort patients experiencing diverticulitis?
    A. Benadryl
    B. Diazepam
    C. Furosemide
    D. Phenergan

_____**172.** Erosion of the gastrointestinal tract caused by gastric acid is termed:
    A. esophageal reflux.
    B. esophagitis.
    C. gastroenteritis.
    D. peptic ulcer.

_____**173.** Common signs and symptoms of Crohn's disease include all of the following **except**:
    A. diarrhea.
    B. recent weight loss.
    C. localized periumbilical pain.
    D. fever.

_____**174.** The artificial replacement of some critical kidney functions is:
   A. dialysate.
   B. hemodialysis.
   C. peritoneal lavage.
   D. renal dialysis.

_____**175.** The pathophysiology of toxic inhalation involves:
   A. bronchoconstriction and dispersal of surfactant.
   B. bronchodilation and destruction of cilia.
   C. irritation, edema, and destruction of alveolar tissue.
   D. pulmonary hypertension, alveolar atelectasis, and destruction of cilia.

_____**176.** All of the following are goals of decontamination **except** to:
   A. enhance elimination of toxin.
   B. reduce absorption of toxin into the body.
   C. reduce intake of toxin.
   D. reduce the elimination of the toxin.

_____**177.** Exposure to all of the following agents is most commonly through ingestion, **except**:
   A. magnesium.
   B. cleaning agents.
   C. cosmetics.
   D. gasoline.

_____**178.** Which of the following questions **is not** important to ask when evaluating a patient who has ingested a toxin?
   A. Have you attempted to induce vomiting?
   B. How much was ingested?
   C. What did you ingest?
   D. What is your height?

_____**179.** Scenario: A patient is complaining of chills, fever, joint pain, and vomiting. Physical examination reveals a 1 cm skin ulceration on the right posterior shoulder, with exudates and a bleb with a white halo. The **best** treatment for this patient should consist of:
   A. calcium chloride 1 gm.
   B. calcium gluconate 0.1 mg/kg.
   C. diazepam 2.5 mg.
   D. supportive management.

_____**180.** Scenario: Your patient has been in jail for five days for driving under the influence and is charged with vehicular manslaughter. The guards have called EMS because the patient is now sweating profusely, is very anxious and unable to sleep, has tremors in his hands and legs, and is afraid that a flying cat is going to eat him. Vitals are pulse of 142, blood pressure of 132/94, and respirations of 34. Dextrostix is 85 mg/dl. Your treatment should consist of:
   A. Thiamine 50 mg.
   B. D50 25 gm.
   C. establishing IV access.
   D. Narcan 2 mg.

_____ **181.** An inadequate number of red blood cells or inadequate hemoglobin within the red blood cells is known as:
  A. anemia.
  B. hyperplasmolysis.
  C. hypoerythrocytosis.
  D. phagocytosis.

_____ **182.** An abnormally high hematocrit that may occur as a result of dehydration is:
  A. erythrocythemia.
  B. hypererythropoiesis.
  C. neutropenia.
  D. polycythemia.

_____ **183.** All of the following environmental factors will exacerbate a preexisting illness **except**:
  A. acute changes in temperature.
  B. high atmospheric pressures.
  C. humidity.
  D. seasonal allergens.

_____ **184.** _____ is freezing of body tissues that results in cellular destruction.
  A. Frostbite
  B. Frostnip
  C. Peripheral tissue hyponecrosis
  D. Trench foot

_____ **185.** In the near-drowning victim, which of the following is a protective mechanism resulting from cold water submersion?
  A. Bradycardia
  B. Mammalian diving reflex
  C. Stimulation of the central nervous system
  D. Vasodilation

_____ **186.** Barotrauma during diving results from:
  A. hyperventilation.
  B. nitrogen narcosis.
  C. rapid ascent.
  D. uncontrolled descent.

_____ **187.** All of the following can help to prevent high altitude illness **except**:
  A. acclimatization.
  B. appropriate sleep.
  C. eating a high carbohydrate diet.
  D. extreme exertion and exercise.

_____ **188.** _____ are microorganisms that reside in the body without ordinarily causing disease.
  A. Normal flora
  B. Opportunistic pathogens
  C. Pathogens
  D. Virulent parasites

_____**189.** Hepatitis E is associated with:
   A. contaminated drinking water.
   B. HBV infection.
   C. HIV.
   D. tuberculosis infection.

_____**190.** All of the following pathogens typically cause meningitis in children **except**:
   A. Haemophilus influenza type B.
   B. Neisseria meningitidis.
   C. Paramyxovirus.
   D. Streptococcus pneumoniae.

_____**191.** The characteristic facial expression seen with tetanus is:
   A. boca satirus.
   B. cheshire risus.
   C. labia sardonicus.
   D. risus sardonicus.

_____**192.** Mononucleosis presents with all of the following signs or symptoms **except**:
   A. enlarged and tender lymph nodes.
   B. fatigue lasting several weeks.
   C. hepatic megaly.
   D. oral discharges.

_____**193.** Lyme disease may result in inflammation of _____ Bell's Palsy.
   A. CN-I
   B. CN-V
   C. CN-VII
   D. CN-XII

_____**194.** A profound sadness or melancholy characterized by diminished interest in daily pleasures, hypersomnia, feelings of helplessness, inability to concentrate, and agitation is:
   A. anxiety.
   B. depression.
   C. phobia.
   D. schizophrenia.

_____**195.** A patient who sustains loss of function in the right arm and leg after an accident, with no apparent medical cause **most likely** has _____ disorder.
   A. conversion
   B. pain
   C. body dismorphic
   D. somatization

_____**196.** The **most common** form of gynecological trauma is:
   A. abdominal trauma.
   B. foreign body trauma.
   C. self-induced abortion.
   D. straddle injury.

_____**197.** Differential diagnosis questions that focus on dysmenorrhea generally would include all of the following **except**:
  A. Do you have any nausea, vomiting, diarrhea, or constipation?
  B. Have you ever been diagnosed with macular degeneration?
  C. Is there any pain during urination?
  D. Is there any unusual vaginal discharge or bleeding?

_____**198.** To prevent under- or over-transfusion of the infant during delivery, the EMS provider should:
  A. milk the umbilical cord.
  B. allow the baby to suckle on the mother's breast.
  C. keep the infant at the level of the vagina.
  D. raise the child above the level of the birth canal.

_____**199.** After the infant is born, EMS personnel should:
  A. allow the afterbirth to deliver naturally.
  B. avoid fundal massage until the placenta is delivered.
  C. pack the vagina with sterile dressings.
  D. pull on the umbilical cord to facilitate delivery of the afterbirth.

_____**200.** Airbags have been introduced to help reduce the injuries received in automobile collisions. With certain age groups, airbags have inflicted serious injury or death. The age group that is **most** susceptible to these injuries is:
  A. geriatric.
  B. pediatric.
  C. adult.
  D. adolescent.

Did you score higher than 80 percent on Examination I-3? Circle Yes or No in ink.

Feedback Step

Now, what do we do with your "yes" and "no" answers given throughout the SAEP process? First, return to any response that has "no" circled. Go back to the highlighted answers for those examination items missed. Read and study the paragraph preceding the location of the answer, as well as the paragraph following the paragraph where the answer is located. This will expand your knowledge base for the missed question, put it in a broader perspective, and improve associative learning. Remember, you are trying to develop mastery of the required knowledge. Scoring 80 percent on an examination is good but it is not mastery performance. To be at the top of your group you must score much higher than 80 percent on your training, promotion, or certification examination.

Carefully review the Summary of Key Rules for Taking an Examination and the Summary of Helpful Hints on the next two pages. Do this review now and at least two additional times prior to taking your next examination.

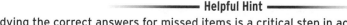

━ Helpful Hint ━

Studying the correct answers for missed items is a critical step in achieving your desired return on effort! The focus of attention is broadened, and new knowledge is often gained by expanding association and contextual learning. During PTS's research and field test, self study during this step of SAEP resulted in gains of 17 points between the first examination administered and the third examination. A gain of 17 points can move you from the lower middle to the top of the list of persons taking a training, promotion, or certification examination. That is a competitive edge and prime example of return on effort in action. Remember: Maximum effort = maximum results!

Summary of Key Rules for Taking an Examination

Rule 1—Examination preparation is not easy. Preparation is 95% perspiration and 5% inspiration.

Rule 2—Follow the steps very carefully. Do not try to reinvent or shortcut the system. It really works just as it was designed to!

Rule 3—Mark with an "X" any examination items for which you guessed the answer. For maximum return on effort, you should also research any answer that you guessed even if you guessed correctly. Find the correct answer, highlight it, and then read the entire paragraph that contains the answer. Be honest and mark all questions on which you guessed. Some examinations have a correction for guessing built into the scoring process. The correction for guessing can reduce your final examination score. If you are guessing, you are not mastering the material.

Rule 4—Read questions twice if you have any misunderstanding, especially if the question contains complex directions or activities.

Rule 5—If you want someone to perform effectively and efficiently on the job, the training and testing program must be aligned to achieve this result.

Rule 6—When preparing examination items for job-specific requirements, the writer must be a subject matter expert with current experience at the level that the technical information is applied.

Rule 7—Good luck = good preparation.

Summary of Helpful Hints

Helpful Hint—Most of the time your first impression is the best. More than 41% of changed answers during PTS's SAEP field test were changed from a right answer to a wrong answer. Another 33% were changed from a wrong answer to another wrong answer. Only 26% of answers were changed from wrong to right. In fact, three participants did not make a perfect score of 100% because they changed one right answer to a wrong one! Think twice before you change your answer. The odds are not in your favor.

Helpful Hint—Researching correct answers is one of the most important activities in SAEP. Locate the correct answer for all missed examination items. Highlight the correct answer. Then read the entire paragraph containing the answer. This will put the answer in context for you and provide important learning by association.

Helpful Hint—Proceed through all missed examination items using the same technique. Reading the entire paragraph improves retention of the information and helps you develop an association with the material and learn the correct answers. This step may sound simple. A major finding during the development and field testing of SAEP was that you learn from your mistakes.

Helpful Hint—Follow each step carefully to realize the best return on effort. Would you consider investing your money in a venture without some chance of earning a return on that investment? Examination preparation is no different. You are investing time and expecting a significant return for that time. If, indeed, time is money, then you are investing money and are due a return on that investment. Doing things right and doing the right things in examination preparation will ensure the maximum return on effort.

Helpful Hint—Try to determine why you selected the wrong answer. Usually something influenced your selection. Focus on the difference between your wrong answer and the correct answer. Carefully read and study the entire paragraph containing the correct answer. Highlight the answer.

Helpful Hint—Studying the correct answers for missed items is a critical step in achieving your desired return on effort! The focus of attention is broadened, and new knowledge is often gained by expanding association and contextual learning. During PTS's research and field test, self-study during this step of SAEP resulted in gains of 17 points between the first examination administered and the third examination. A gain of 17 points can move you from the lower middle to the top of the list of persons taking a training, promotion, or certification examination. That is a competitive edge and a prime example of return on effort in action. Remember: Maximum effort = maximum results!

PHASE II

How Examination Developers Think—Getting Inside Their Heads

Now that you've finished the examination practice, this phase will assist you in understanding and applying examination-taking skills. Developing your knowledge of how examination professionals think and prepare examinations is not cheating. Most serious examination takers have spent many hours reviewing various examinations to gain an insight into the technology used to develop them. It is a demanding technology when used properly. You probably already know this if you have prepared examination items and administered them in your EMS department.

Phase II will not cover all the ways and means of examination-item writing. Examination-item writers use far too many techniques to cover adequately in this book. Instead, the focus here is on key techniques that will help you achieve a better score on your examination.

How are examination items derived?

Professional examination-item writers use three basic techniques to derive examination items from text or technical reference materials: verbatim, deduction, and inference.

The most common technique is to take examination items verbatim from materials in the reference list. This technique doesn't work well for mastering information, however. The verbatim form of testing encourages rote learning—that is, simply memorizing the material. The results of this type of learning are not long-lasting, nor are they appropriate for learning and retaining the critical knowledge you must have for on-the-job performance. Consequently, SAEP doesn't create the majority of examination questions covering the DOT National Standard Curriculum using the verbatim technique.

Professional examination-item writers tend to use verbatim testing at the very basic level of job classifications. A first responder, for instance, is expected to learn many basic facts. At this level, verbatim examination items can be justified.

In the higher ranks of Emergency Medical Services other methods are more beneficial and productive for mastering higher cognitive knowledge and skills. At the higher cognitive levels of an occupation, such as EMS Supervisor, examination development will therefore rely on other means. The most important technique at the higher cognitive levels is using deduction as the basis for examination items. This technique requires logic and analytical skills and often requires the examination taker to read materials several times to answer the examination item. It is not, then, a matter of simply repeating the information that results in a verbatim answer.

At the first responder level, most activities are carefully supervised by a more experienced technician or company officer. At this level, the responder is expected to closely follow commands and is encouraged not to use deductive reasoning that can lead to "freelance" responder tactics. As one progresses to a higher level job and gains experience, deductive reasoning and skills are developed and applied. Most of these skills are related to personal safety and the safety of those on the scene. Most sizeups and strategies are developed and passed from the officers on the scene to the first responders.

——————— **Rule 5** ———————

If you want someone to perform effectively and efficiently on the job, the training and testing program must be aligned to achieve this result.

Rule #5 is paramount for first responders. Effective and efficient first responders are able to receive incident commands, follow instructions, and perform their tasks as safely and as rapidly as they can. There are limited opportunities for first responders to do much else, because they are the first line of action at the emergency scene.

Consider the following example of deductive reasoning: an incident call is received from the telecommunicator stating that an infant has a high temperature and is convulsing. Just this amount of information should cause the first responder to immediately plan the response, conduct sizeup activities, and review infant care procedures en route. Some of these deductive responses will have you focus on the infant's age, past medical history, location, access, and many other possible factors. If you have an EMT or Paramedic background, a list of several items could be deduced that would expedite an efficient and effective response to the incident.

You can probably think of many first responder tasks and circumstances that rely on deductive reasoning. The more you gain experience on the emergency scene as a Paramedic, the more you will get to practice deductive reasoning and inference from emergency data, and the more efficient and effective you will become whether it is clearing an airway or attending to the emergency needs of an infant.

Legendary football coach Vince Lombardi was once asked about the precision performance of his offensive and defensive teams. It was suggested that Lombardi must spend a lot of time on the practice field to achieve those results. Lombardi responded, "Practice doesn't make perfect, only perfect practice makes perfect." This is exactly what is required to be an outstanding examination taker. Most people don't perfectly practice examination-taking skills.

A third technique used by the professional examination-item writers is to rely on inference or implied answers to develop examination items. Inference requires contrasting, comparing, analyzing, evaluating, and other high-level cognitive skills. Tables, charts, graphs, and other instruments for presenting data provide excellent means for deriving inference-based examination items. Implied answers are based on logic. They rely on your ability to use logical processes or series of facts to arrive at a plausible answer.

For example, recent data supplied by the National Fire Protection Association stated that heart attacks remain the leading cause of death for fire service personnel. Other NFPA-supplied data indicated that strains and sprains are the leading cause of injuries on the job. Several inferences can be made from these relatively simple statements. A safety officer can apply the results of the NFPA to his or her own personnel and use the information as a trigger for checking on personnel, conducting surveys, reviewing accident records, and comparing the results with actual experience. Is that particular EMS division doing better or worse in terms of these important health issues? Are the first responders getting the right exercise? Are they diligent in keeping the vehicles, facilities, and emergency scene free from the activities that may lead to strains and sprains? The basic inference here is that any particular organization may be similar or different in some ways from the generalized data.

Sometimes it may be difficult to find an answer to an examination item because it is measuring your ability to make deductions and draw inferences from the technical materials.

How are examination items written and validated?

Once the pertinent information is identified and the technique for writing an examination item selected, the professional examination-item writer will prepare a draft. The draft examination item is then referenced to specific technical information such as a textbook, manufacturer's manual, or other related technical information. If the information is derived from a job-based requirement, then it should also be validated by job incumbents (i.e., those who are actually performing in the occupation at the specific level of the required knowledge).

Rule 6

When preparing examination items for job-specific requirements, the writer must be a subject matter expert with current experience at the level where the technical information is applied.

Rule #6 ensures that the examination item has a basic level of job content validity. The final level of job content validity is determined by using committees or surveys of job incumbents who certify the information to be current and required on the job. The information must be in a category of "need to know" or "must know" to be considered job relevant. The technical information must be accurate. Because subject matter experts do need basic training in examination-item writing, it is recommended that a professional in examination technology be part of the review process so that basic rules and guidelines of the industry are followed.

Finally, the examination items must be field tested. Once this testing is complete, statistical and analytical tools are available to help revise and improve the examination items. These techniques and tools go well beyond the scope of this *Exam Prep* book. Professionals are available to conduct these data analyses, and their services should be used.

Good Practices in Examination-Item and Examination Development

The most reliable examinations are objective. That is, each question has only one answer that is accepted by members of the occupation. This objective quality permits fair and equitable examinations. The most popular types of objective examination items are multiple choice, true/false, matching, and completion (fill in the blanks).

Valid and reliable job-relevant examinations for the Emergency Medical Service industry must satisfy 10 rules:

1. They do not contain trick questions.
2. They are short and easy to read, using language and terms appropriate to the target examination population.
3. They are supported with technical references, validation information, and data on their difficulty, discrimination, and other item analysis statistics.
4. They are formatted to meet recognized testing standards and examples.
5. They focus on the "need to know" and "must know" aspects of the job.
6. They are fair and objective.
7. They are not based on obscure and trivial knowledge and skills.
8. They can be easily defended in terms of job-content requirements.
9. They meet national and other professional job qualification standards.
10. They demonstrate their usefulness as part of a comprehensive testing program, including written, oral, and performance examination items.

The primary challenges of job-relevant examinations relate to their currency and validity. Careful recording of data, technical reference sources, and the examination writer's qualifications are important. Examinations that affect someone's ability to be promoted, certified, or licensed, as well as to complete training that leads to a job, have exacting requirements both in published documents and in the laws of the land.

Three Common Myths of Examination Construction

1. **Myth:** If in doubt about the answer for a multiple-choice examination item, select the longest answer in a multiple choice examination item.

   Reality—Professional examination-item writers use short answers as correct ones at an equal or higher percentage than longer answers. Remember, there are usually choices A-D. That leaves three other possibilities for the correct answer other than the longest one. Statistically speaking, the longest answer is less likely to be correct.

2. **Myth:** If in doubt about the answer in a multiple-choice examination item, select "C".

   Reality—Computer technology and examination-item banking permit multiple versions of examinations to be developed simultaneously. This is typically achieved by moving the correct answer to different locations (for example, version 1 will have the correct answer in the "C" position, version 2 in the "D" position, and so forth).

3. **Myth:** Watch for errors in singular examination-item stems with plural choices in the A-D answers, or vice versa.

   Reality—Most computer-based programs have spelling and grammar checking utilities. If this mistake occurs, an editing error is the probable cause and usually has nothing to do with detecting the right answer.

Some Things That Work

1. Two to three days before your examination, review the examination items you missed in SAEP. Read those highlighted answers and the entire paragraph one more time.

2. During the examination, carefully read the examination item twice. Once you have selected your answer, read the examination item and answer together. This technique can prompt you to recall information that you studied during your *Exam Prep* activities.

3. Apply what you learned in SAEP. Eliminate as many distracters as possible to improve your chance of answering the question correctly.

4. Pace yourself. Know how much time you have to take the examination. If an examination item is requiring too much time, write its number down and continue with the next examination item. Often, a later examination item will trigger your memory and make the examination item seem easier to answer. (For a time pacing strategy, see the Examination Pacing Table at the end of Phase III.)

5. Don't panic if you don't know some examination items. Leave them to answer later. The most important thing is to finish the examination, because there may be several examination items at the end of the examination that you do know.

6. As time runs out for taking the examination, don't panic. Concentrate on answering those difficult examination items that you skipped.

7. Double-check your answer sheets to make sure you haven't accidentally left an answer blank.

8. Once you complete the examination, return to the difficult examination items. Often, while taking an examination, other examination items will cause you to remember or associate those answers with the difficult examination-item answers. The longer the examination, the more likely you will be to gather information needed to answer more difficult examination items.

There are many other helpful hints that can be used to improve your examination-taking skills. If you want to research the materials on how to take examinations and raise your final score, go to the local library, a bookstore, or the Web for additional resources. The main reason we developed SAEP is to provide practice and help you develop examination-taking skills you can use throughout your life.

PHASE III

The Basics of Mental and Physical Preparation

Mental Preparation—I Can Get My Head Ready!

The two most common mental blocks to examination taking are examination anxiety and fear of failure. In the Emergency Medical Service these feelings can create significant performance barriers. Overcoming severe conditions may require some professional psychological assistance, which is beyond the scope of this *Exam Prep* book.

The root cause of feelings of examination anxiety and fear of failure is often a lack of self-confidence. SAEP was designed to help improve your self-confidence by providing evidence of your mastery of the material on the examination. Look at your scores as you progress through Phase I. Review your Personal Progress Plotter; it will help you gain confidence in your knowledge of the EMT-Paramedic curriculum. Look at your Personal Progress Plotter the day before your scheduled examination and experience renewed confidence.

Let's examine the meaning of anxiety. Knowing what it is will help you deal with it at examination time. According to *Webster's Dictionary*, anxiety is "uneasiness and distress about future uncertainties." Many of us have real anxiety about taking examinations, and it is a natural response for some, often prefaced by such questions like these: Am I ready for this? Do I have a good idea of what will be on the examination? Will I make the lowest score? Will John Doe score higher than me?

These questions and concerns are normal. Remember that hundreds of people have gone through SAEP with an average gain of 17 points in their scores. The preparation process will help you maintain your self-confidence. Once again, review the evidence in your Personal Progress Plotter to see what you have accomplished.

Fear, according to *Webster's Dictionary*, is "alarm and agitation caused by the expectation or realization of danger." It is a normal reaction to examinations. To deal with it, first, analyze the degree of fear you may be experiencing several days before the examination date. Then focus on the positive experiences you had as you finished SAEP. Putting fear in perspective by using positives to eliminate or minimize it is a very important examination-taking skill. The more you focus on your positive accomplishments in mastering the materials, the less fear you will experience.

If fear and anxiety persist, even after taking steps to build your confidence, you may want to get some professional assistance. Do it now! Don't wait until the week before the examination. There may be real issues that a professional can help you deal with to overcome these feelings. Hypnosis and other forms of treatment have been found to be very helpful. Consult with an expert in this area.

Physical Preparation—Am I Really Ready?

Physical preparation is the element that is probably most ignored in examination preparation. In the Emergency Medical Service, examinations are often given at locations away from home. If this is the case, you need to be especially careful of key physical concerns. More will be said about that later.

In general, following these helpful hints will help you concentrate, enhance your examination performance, and add points to your score.

1. Do not "cram" for the examination. This factor was found to be first in importance during PTS's field test of SAEP. Cramming results in examination anxiety, adds to confusion, and tends to lessen the effectiveness of examination-taking skills you possess. Avoid cramming!

2. Get a normal night's rest. It may even be wise to take a day off before the examination to rest. Do not schedule an all-night shift right before your examination.

3. Avoid taking excessive stimulants or medications that inhibit your thinking processes. Eat at least three well-balanced meals before the day of the examination. It is a good practice to carry a balanced energy bar (not candy) and a bottle of water into the examination area. Examination anxiety and fear can cause a dry mouth, which can lead to further aggravation. Nibbling on the energy bar also has a settling effect and supplies some "brain food."

4. If the examination is taking place at an out-of-town location, do the following:
   - Avoid a "night out with friends." Lack of rest, partying, and fatigue are major examination performance killers.
   - Check your room carefully. Eliminate things that may aggravate you, interfere with your rest, or cause any discomfort. If the mattress isn't good, the pillows are horrible, or the room has an unpleasant odor, change rooms or even hotels.
   - Wake up in plenty of time to take a relaxing shower or soaking bath. Do not put yourself in a "rush" mode. Things should be carefully planned so that you arrive at the examination site ahead of time, calm, and collected.

5. Listen to the examination proctor. The proctor usually has rules that you must follow. Important instructions and directions are usually given. Ask clarifying questions immediately and listen to the response to questions raised by the other examination takers. Most examination environments are carefully controlled and may not permit questions you raise that are covered in the proctor's comments or deal with the technical content in the examination itself. Be attentive, focus, and succeed.

6. Remain calm and breathe. Pace yourself. Apply your examination-taking skills learned during SAEP.

7. Remember the analogy of an examination as a competitive event. If you want to gain a competitive edge, carefully follow all phases of SAEP. This process has yielded outstanding results in the past and will do so for you.

Time Management During Examinations

The following table will help you pace yourself during an examination. You should become familiar with the table and be able to construct your own when you are in the examination room and getting ready to start the examination process. This effort will take a few minutes, but it will make a tremendous contribution to your time management during the examination.

Here is how the table works. First you divide the examination time into 6 equal parts. If you have 3½ hours (210 minutes) for the examination, then each of the six time parts contains 35 minutes (210 ÷ 6 = 35 minutes). Now divide the number of examination items by 5. For example, if the examination has 150 examination items, 150 ÷ 5 = 30. Now, with the math done, we can set up a table that tells you approximately how many examination items you should answer in 35 minutes (the equal time divisions). You should be on or near examination item 30 at the end of the first 35 minutes and so forth. Notice that we divided the number of examination items by 5 and the time available by 6. This extra time block of 35 minutes is used to double-check your answer sheet, focus on difficult questions, and to calm your nerves. This technique will work wonders for your stress level, and yes, it will improve your examination score.

Examination Pacing Table

Time for Examination	Minutes for 6 Equal Time Parts	Number of Examination Items	Examination Items per Time Part	Time for Examination Review
210 minutes (3.5 hours)	35 minutes	150	30 (number of examination items to be answered)	35 minutes (chilling and double-checking examination)
276 minutes (4.6 hours)	46 minutes	200	40 (number of examination items to be answered)	46 minutes (chilling and double-checking examination)

The Examination Pacing Table can be altered by adjusting the time and examination item variables, as either may change in the real examination environment. For instance, if the time changes, adjust the amount of time available to answer the examination items in each of the five time blocks. If the examination item numbers increase or decrease, adjust the number of examination items to be answered in the time blocks.

Take some precautions when using this time management strategy:

1. Do not panic if you run a few minutes behind in each time block. This time management strategy should not stress you while you are using it. Most people tend to pick up their pace as they move into the examination.
2. During the examination, carefully mark or note examination items that you need to return to during your review time block. This will help you expedite your examination completion check.
3. Do not be afraid to ask for more time to complete your examination. In most cases, the time limit is flexible or should be.
4. Double-check your answer sheet to make sure that you didn't leave blank responses and that you didn't double-mark answers. Double-markings are most often counted as wrong answers. Make sure that any erasures are made cleanly. Caution: When you change your answer, make sure that you really want to do so. The odds are not in your favor unless something on the examination really influenced the change.

APPENDIX A

Examination I-1 Answer Key

Directions
Follow these steps carefully for completing the feedback part of SAEP:

1. After calculating your score, look up the answers for the examination items you missed as well as those on which you guessed, even if you guessed correctly. If you are guessing, it means the answer is not perfectly clear. In this process, we are committed to making you as knowledgeable as possible.

2. Enter the number of missed and guessed examination items in the blanks on your Personal Progress Plotter.

3. Highlight the answer in the reference materials. Read the paragraph preceding and the paragraph following the one in which the correct answer is located. Enter the paragraph number and page number next to the guessed or missed examination item on your examination. Count any part of a paragraph at the beginning of the page as one paragraph until you reach the paragraph containing your highlighted answer. This step will help you locate and review your missed and guessed examination items later in the process. It is essential to learning the material in context and by association. These learning techniques (context/association) are the very backbone of the SAEP approach.

4. Once you have completed the feedback part, you may proceed to the next examination.

1. Reference: DOT Standard 1-1.1(A)
   Brady, *Essentials of Paramedic Care*, 1st Edition, pages 1044-1050 and 1054.
   Answer: B

2. Reference: DOT 1-1.1(c)
   Brady, *Essentials of Paramedic Care*, 1st Edition, page 17.
   Mosby, *Paramedic Textbook*, Revised 2nd Edition, page 15.
   Answer: A

3. Reference: DOT 1-1.1(b)
   Brady, *Essentials of Paramedic Care*, 1st Edition, page 17.
   Mosby, *Paramedic Textbook*, Revised 2nd Edition, page 15.
   Answer: B

4. Reference: DOT 1-1.1(d)
   Brady, *Essentials of Paramedic Care*, 1st Edition, page 17.
   Mosby, *Paramedic Textbook*, Revised 2nd Edition, page 15.
   Answer: C

5. Reference: DOT 1-1.1(e)
Brady, *Essentials of Paramedic Care*, 1st Edition, page 17.
Mosby, *Paramedic Textbook*, Revised 2nd Edition, page 15.
Answer: D

6. Reference: DOT 1-2.1
Brady, *Essentials of Paramedic Care*, 1st Edition, page 33.
Mosby, *Paramedic Textbook*, Revised 2nd Edition, page 34.
Answer: D

7. Reference: DOT 1-2.1
Brady, *Essentials of Paramedic Care*, 1st Edition, page 33.
Mosby, *Paramedic Textbook*, Revised 2nd Edition, page 34.
Answer: C

8. Reference: DOT 1-2.2
Brady, *Essentials of Paramedic Care*, 1st Edition, page 33.
Mosby, *Paramedic Textbook*, Revised 2nd Edition, pages 34-35.
Answer: D

9. Reference: DOT 1-3.1
Brady, *Essentials of Paramedic Care*, 1st Edition, page 856.
Answer: B

10. Reference: DOT 1-4.1
Brady, *Essentials of Paramedic Care*, 1st Edition, page 79.
Mosby, *Paramedic Textbook*, Revised 2nd Edition, page 67.
Answer: C

11. Reference: DOT 1-4.1
Brady, *Essentials of Paramedic Care*, 1st Edition, page 74.
Mosby, *Paramedic Textbook*, Revised 2nd Edition, page 67.
Answer: A

12. Reference: DOT 1-4.28
Brady, *Essentials of Paramedic Care*, 1st Edition, page 93.
Mosby, *Paramedic Textbook*, Revised 2nd Edition, page 522.
Answer: B

13. Reference: DOT 1-4.3
Brady, *Essentials of Paramedic Care*, 1st Edition, page 75.
Mosby, *Paramedic Textbook*, Revised 2nd Edition, page 68.
Answer: C

14. Reference: DOT 1-5.1
Brady, *Essentials of Paramedic Care*, 1st Edition, page 60.
Mosby, *Paramedic Textbook*, Revised 2nd Edition, page 91.
Answer: C

15. Reference: DOT 1-6.1
Brady, *Essentials of Paramedic Care*, 1st Edition, page 265.
Mosby, *Paramedic Textbook*, Revised 2nd Edition, page 203.
Answer: A

16. Reference: DOT 1-6
Brady, *Essentials of Paramedic Care*, 1st Edition, page 266.
Mosby, *Paramedic Textbook*, Revised 2nd Edition, page 203.
Answer: D

17. Reference: DOT 1-6
Brady, *Essentials of Paramedic Care*, 1st Edition, page 266.
Mosby, *Paramedic Textbook*, Revised 2nd Edition, page 203.
Answer: C

18. Reference: DOT 1-6.1
Brady, *Essentials of Paramedic Care*, 1st Edition, page 265.
Mosby, *Paramedic Textbook*, Revised 2nd Edition, page 203.
Answer: B

19. Reference: DOT 1-6.1
Brady, *Essentials of Paramedic Care*, 1st Edition, page 266.
Mosby, *Paramedic Textbook*, Revised 2nd Edition, page 204.
Answer: B

20. Reference: DOT 1-7.2
Brady, *Essentials of Paramedic Care*, 1st Edition, page 341.
Mosby, *Paramedic Textbook*, Revised 2nd Edition, page 235.
Answer: D

21. Reference: DOT 1-7.2
Brady, *Essentials of Paramedic Care*, 1st Edition, page 341.
Mosby, *Paramedic Textbook*, Revised 2nd Edition, page 234.
Answer: B

22. Reference: DOT 1-7.3
Brady, *Essentials of Paramedic Care*, 1st Edition, page 341.
Mosby, *Paramedic Textbook*, Revised 2nd Edition, page 234.
Answer: C

23. Reference: DOT 1-7.24
Brady, *Essentials of Paramedic Care*, 1st Edition, page 382.
Mosby, *Paramedic Textbook*, Revised 2nd Edition, page 879.
Answer: B

24. Reference: DOT 1-7.5
Brady, *Essentials of Paramedic Care*, 1st Edition, page 341.
Mosby, *Paramedic Textbook*, Revised 2nd Edition, page 235.
Answer: C

25. Reference: DOT 1-7.7
Brady, *Essentials of Paramedic Care*, 1st Edition, page 343.
Mosby, *Paramedic Textbook*, Revised 2nd Edition, page 236.
Answer: C

26. Reference: DOT 1-8.1
Brady, *Essentials of Paramedic Care*, 1st Edition, pages 418-420.
Answer: D

27. Reference: DOT 1-8.6

Brady, *Essentials of Paramedic Care*, 1st Edition, page 491.
Mosby, *Paramedic Textbook*, Revised 2nd Edition, page 309.
Answer: B

28. Reference: DOT 1-8.6

Brady, *Essentials of Paramedic Care*, 1st Edition, pages 489 and 493.
Mosby, *Paramedic Textbook*, Revised 2nd Edition, page 309.
Answer: B

29. Reference: DOT 1-8.5

Brady, *Essentials of Paramedic Care*, 1st Edition, pages 494-495.
Mosby, *Paramedic Textbook*, Revised 2nd Edition, page 312.
Answer: C

30. Reference: DOT 1-8.5

Brady, *Essentials of Paramedic Care*, 1st Edition, page 494.
Mosby, *Paramedic Textbook*, Revised 2nd Edition, page 312.
Answer: B

31. Reference: DOT 1-8.3

Brady, *Essentials of Paramedic Care*, 1st Edition, pages 487-488.
Mosby, *Paramedic Textbook*, Revised 2nd Edition, page 306.
Answer: C

32. Reference: DOT 1-9.1

Brady, *Essentials of Paramedic Care*, 1st Edition, page 575.
Mosby, *Paramedic Textbook*, Revised 2nd Edition, page 345.
Answer: C

33. Reference: DOT 1-9.2

Brady, *Essentials of Paramedic Care*, 1st Edition, page 575.
Answer: D

34. Reference: DOT 1-10.1

Brady, *Essentials of Paramedic Care*, 1st Edition, page 322.
Answer: B

35. Reference: DOT 1-10.8

Brady, *Essentials of Paramedic Care*, 1st Edition, page 335.
Answer: A

36. Reference: DOT 2-1.10

Brady, *Essentials of Paramedic Care*, 1st Edition, page 238.
Mosby, *Paramedic Textbook*, Revised 2nd Edition, page 374.
Answer: B

37. Reference: DOT 2-1.78

Brady, *Essentials of Paramedic Care*, 1st Edition, page 498.
Mosby, *Paramedic Textbook*, Revised 2nd Edition, page 378.
Answer: C

38. Reference: DOT 2-1.2
Brady, *Essentials of Paramedic Care*, 1st Edition, page 508.
Answer: C

39. Reference: DOT 2-1.3
Brady, *Essentials of Paramedic Care*, 1st Edition, page 227.
Mosby, *Paramedic Textbook*, Revised 2nd Edition, pages 155-156.
Answer: D

40. Reference: DOT 2-1.3
Brady, *Essentials of Paramedic Care*, 1st Edition, page 227.
Mosby, *Paramedic Textbook*, Revised 2nd Edition, page 156.
Answer: A

41. Reference: DOT 2-1.12
Brady, *Essentials of Paramedic Care*, 1st Edition, page 237.
Mosby, *Paramedic Textbook*, Revised 2nd Edition, page 374.
Answer: D

42. Reference: DOT 2-1.73
Brady, *Essentials of Paramedic Care*, 1st Edition, page 507.
Mosby, *Paramedic Textbook*, Revised 2nd Edition, pages 416-417.
Answer: B

43. Reference: DOT 2-1.17
Brady, *Essentials of Paramedic Care*, 1st Edition, page 239.
Mosby, *Paramedic Textbook*, Revised 2nd Edition, pages 376-377.
Answer: A

44. Reference: DOT 2-1.11
Brady, *Essentials of Paramedic Care*, 1st Edition, page 508.
Answer: A

45. Reference: DOT 2-1.4
Brady, *Essentials of Paramedic Care*, 1st Edition, page 227.
Mosby, *Paramedic Textbook*, Revised 2nd Edition, pages 155-156.
Answer: B

46. Reference: DOT 3-1.1
Brady, *Essentials of Paramedic Care*, 1st Edition, page 592.
Mosby, *Paramedic Textbook*, Revised 2nd Edition, page 433.
Answer: C

47. Reference: DOT 3-2.1
Brady, *Essentials of Paramedic Care*, 1st Edition, page 610.
Mosby, Paramedic Textbook, Revised 2nd Edition, page 443.
Answer: B

48. Reference: DOT 3-2.2
Brady, *Essentials of Paramedic Care*, 1st Edition, page 611.
Mosby, *Paramedic Textbook*, Revised 2nd Edition, page 443.
Answer: D

49. Reference: DOT 3-2.2
Brady, *Essentials of Paramedic Care*, 1st Edition, page 611.
Mosby, *Paramedic Textbook*, Revised 2nd Edition, page 444.
Answer: A

50. Reference: DOT 3-2.2
Brady, *Essentials of Paramedic Care*, 1st Edition, page 612.
Mosby, *Paramedic Textbook*, Revised 2nd Edition, page 444.
Answer: C

51. Reference: DOT 3-2.3
Brady, *Essentials of Paramedic Care*, 1st Edition, page 678.
Mosby, *Paramedic Textbook*, Revised 2nd Edition, page 448.
Answer: A

52. Reference: DOT 3-2.3
Brady, *Essentials of Paramedic Care*, 1st Edition, page 677.
Mosby, *Paramedic Textbook*, Revised 2nd Edition, page 447.
Answer: A

53. Reference: DOT 3-3.1
Brady, *Essentials of Paramedic Care*, 1st Edition, page 702.
Answer: D

54. Reference: DOT 3-3.2
Brady, *Essentials of Paramedic Care*, 1st Edition, page 705.
Mosby, *Paramedic Textbook*, Revised 2nd Edition, page 1455.
Answer: D

55. Reference: DOT 3-3.3
Brady, *Essentials of Paramedic Care*, 1st Edition, pages 703-704.
Mosby, *Paramedic Textbook*, Revised 2nd Edition, page 1123.
Answer: B

56. Reference: DOT 3-3.5
Brady, *Essentials of Paramedic Care*, 1st Edition, page 705.
Mosby, *Paramedic Textbook*, Revised 2nd Edition, pages 1455–1456.
Answer: D

57. Reference: DOT 3-3.5
Brady, *Essentials of Paramedic Care*, 1st Edition, page 705.
Mosby, *Paramedic Textbook*, Revised 2nd Edition, page 1457.
Answer: B

58. Reference: DOT 3-3.76
Brady, *Essentials of Paramedic Care*, 1st Edition, page 711.
Answer: C

59. Reference: DOT 3-4.1
Brady, *Essentials of Paramedic Care*, 1st Edition, page 758.
Answer: B

60. Reference: DOT 3-4.2
Brady, *Essentials of Paramedic Care*, 1st Edition, page 758.
Answer: A

61. Reference: DOT 3-5.24
Brady, *Essentials of Paramedic Care*, 1st Edition, page 778.
Answer: C

62. Reference: DOT 3-5.22
Brady, *Essentials of Paramedic Care*, 1st Edition, page 772.
Answer: A

63. Reference: DOT 3-5.1
Brady, *Essentials of Paramedic Care*, 1st Edition, page 772.
Answer: B

64. Reference: DOT 3-6.10 and 3-6.6
Brady, *Essentials of Paramedic Care*, 1st Edition, page 792.
Mosby, *Paramedic Textbook*, Revised 2nd Edition, page 520.
Answer: C

65. Reference: DOT 3-6.18
Brady, *Essentials of Paramedic Care*, 1st Edition, page 789.
Mosby, *Paramedic Textbook*, Revised 2nd Edition, page 515.
Answer: C

66. Reference: DOT 3-6.18, 3-6.19, and 3-6.7
Brady, *Essentials of Paramedic Care*, 1st Edition, pages 516, 520, and 521.
Mosby, *Paramedic Textbook*, Revised 2nd Edition, page 521.
Answer: B

67. Reference: DOT 3-6.22 and 3-6.18
Brady, *Essentials of Paramedic Care*, 1st Edition, page 790.
Mosby, *Paramedic Textbook*, Revised 2nd Edition, page 515.
Answer: A

68. Reference: DOT 4-1.10
Brady, *Essentials of Paramedic Care*, 1st Edition, page 1139.
Answer: C

69. Reference: DOT 4-1.6 and 4-1.5
Brady, *Essentials of Paramedic Care*, 1st Edition, page 849.
Answer: A

70. Reference: DOT 4-1.10
Brady, *Essentials of Paramedic Care*, 1st Edition, page 851.
Answer: C

71. Reference: DOT 4-1.11
Brady, *Essentials of Paramedic Care*, 1st Edition, page 850.
Answer: D

72. Reference: DOT 4-2.16
Brady, *Essentials of Paramedic Care*, 1st Edition, page 879.
Answer: D

73. Reference: DOT 4-2.26
Brady, *Essentials of Paramedic Care*, 1st Edition, page 177.
Mosby, *Paramedic Textbook*, Revised 2nd Edition, page 759.
Answer: C

74. Reference: DOT 4-2.2
Brady, *Essentials of Paramedic Care*, 1st Edition, page 218.
Answer: D

75. Reference: DOT 4-3.1
Brady, *Essentials of Paramedic Care*, 1st Edition, page 912.
Answer: D

76. Reference: DOT 4-3.2(B)
Brady, *Essentials of Paramedic Care*, 1st Edition, page 118.
Answer: C

77. Reference: DOT 4-3.3
Brady, *Essentials of Paramedic Care*, 1st Edition, page 912.
Mosby, *Paramedic Textbook*, Revised 2nd Edition, page 113.
Answer: D

78. Reference: DOT 4-4.1
Brady, *Essentials of Paramedic Care*, 1st Edition, page 118.
Mosby, *Paramedic Textbook*, Revised 2nd Edition, pages 113-114 and 573.
Answer: D

79. Reference: DOT 4-4.2
Brady, *Essentials of Paramedic Care*, 1st Edition, page 954.
Answer: C

80. Reference: DOT 4-4.3
Brady, *Essentials of Paramedic Care*, 1st Edition, page 955.
Mosby, *Paramedic Textbook*, Revised 2nd Edition, page 605.
Answer: D

81. Reference: DOT 4-5.35 and 4-5.37
Brady, *Essentials of Paramedic Care*, 1st Edition, page 1026.
Answer: C

82. Reference: DOT 4-5.1
Brady, *Essentials of Paramedic Care*, 1st Edition, page 1040.
Answer: B

83. Reference: DOT 4-5.35
Brady, *Essentials of Paramedic Care*, 1st Edition, page 154.
Answer: D

84. Reference: DOT 4-6.2
Brady, *Essentials of Paramedic Care*, 1st Edition, page 855.
Answer: C

85. Reference: DOT 4-6.3
Brady, *Essentials of Paramedic Care*, 1st Edition, page 1069.
Mosby, *Paramedic Textbook*, Revised 2nd Edition, page 657.
Answer: B

86. Reference: DOT 4-6.2(G) and 4-6.2(H)
Brady, *Essentials of Paramedic Care*, 1st Edition, page 177.
Mosby, *Paramedic Textbook*, Revised 2nd Edition, page 129.
Answer: C

87. Reference: DOT 4-7.14 and 4-1.9
Brady, *Essentials of Paramedic Care*, 1st Edition, page 835.
Mosby, *Paramedic Textbook*, Revised 2nd Edition, page 538.
Answer: D

88. Reference: DOT 4-7.21 and 4-7.21(A)
Brady, *Essentials of Paramedic Care*, 1st Edition, pages 838-839.
Answer: A

89. Reference: DOT 4-7.1
Brady, *Essentials of Paramedic Care*, 1st Edition, page 1100.
Answer: B

90. Reference: DOT 4-8.1
Brady, *Essentials of Paramedic Care*, 1st Edition, page 1134.
Mosby, *Paramedic Textbook*, Revised 2nd Edition, page 527.
Answer: B

91. Reference: DOT 4-8.6
Brady, *Essentials of Paramedic Care*, 1st Edition, page 1137.
Mosby, *Paramedic Textbook*, Revised 2nd Edition, page 702.
Answer: A

92. Reference: DOT 4-9.1
Brady, *Essentials of Paramedic Care*, 1st Edition, page 988.
Mosby, *Paramedic Textbook*, Revised 2nd Edition, page 527.
Answer: C

93. Reference: DOT 4-9.2
Brady, *Essentials of Paramedic Care*, 1st Edition, page 130.
Mosby, *Paramedic Textbook*, Revised 2nd Edition, page 125.
Answer: A

94. Reference: DOT 1-1.15, 1-1.16
Brady, *Essentials of Paramedic Care*, 1st Edition, page 1022.
Mosby, *Paramedic Textbook*, Revised 2nd Edition, page 16.
Answer: B

95. Reference: DOT 4-9.2

Brady, *Essentials of Paramedic Care*, 1st Edition, page 131.
Answer: C

96. Reference: DOT 5-1.2

Brady, *Essentials of Paramedic Care*, 1st Edition, pages 226 and 229.
Mosby, *Paramedic Textbook*, Revised 2nd Edition, pages 157-158.
Answer: D

97. Reference: DOT 5-1.2

Brady, *Essentials of Paramedic Care*, 1st Edition, page 228.
Mosby, *Paramedic Textbook*, Revised 2nd Edition, page 155.
Answer: C

98. Reference: DOT 5-1.2

Brady, *Essentials of Paramedic Care*, 1st Edition, page 229.
Mosby, *Paramedic Textbook*, Revised 2nd Edition, page 155.
Answer: C

99. Reference: DOT 5-1.2

Brady, *Essentials of Paramedic Care*, 1st Edition, page 228.
Mosby, *Paramedic Textbook*, Revised 2nd Edition, pages 155 and 1565.
Answer: B

100. Reference: DOT 5-1.6

Brady, *Essentials of Paramedic Care*, 1st Edition, page 523.
Mosby, *Paramedic Textbook*, Revised 2nd Edition, page 411.
Answer: A

101. Reference: DOT 5-2.1

Brady, *Essentials of Paramedic Care*, 1st Edition, page 1201.
Answer: B

102. Reference: DOT 5-2.3

Brady, *Essentials of Paramedic Care*, 1st Edition, page 1201.
Mosby, *Paramedic Textbook*, Revised 2nd Edition, page 754.
Answer: B

103. Reference: DOT 5-2.3

Brady, *Essentials of Paramedic Care*, 1st Edition, page 1201.
Mosby, *Paramedic Textbook*, Revised 2nd Edition, page 754.
Answer: D

104. Reference: DOT 5-2.4

Brady, *Essentials of Paramedic Care*, 1st Edition, page 207.
Mosby, *Paramedic Textbook*, Revised 2nd Edition, page 148.
Answer: B

105. Reference: DOT 5-2.4

Brady, *Essentials of Paramedic Care*, 1st Edition, page 1202.
Mosby, *Paramedic Textbook*, Revised 2nd Edition, page 149.
Answer: C

106. Reference: DOT 5-2.5
Brady, *Essentials of Paramedic Care*, 1st Edition, page 210.
Mosby, *Paramedic Textbook*, Revised 2nd Edition, page 884.
Answer: C

107. Reference: DOT 5-2.5
Brady, *Essentials of Paramedic Care*, 1st Edition, pages 218 and 220.
Mosby, *Paramedic Textbook*, Revised 2nd Edition, pages 152 and 1596.
Answer: D

108. Reference: DOT 5-2.6
Brady, *Essentials of Paramedic Care*, 1st Edition, page 218.
Answer: A

109. Reference: DOT 5-2.7
Brady, *Essentials of Paramedic Care*, 1st Edition, page 222.
Mosby, *Paramedic Textbook*, Revised 2nd Edition, page 756.
Answer: D

110. Reference: DOT 5-2.8
Brady, *Essentials of Paramedic Care*, 1st Edition, pages 222 and 2069.
Answer: D

111. Reference: DOT 5-2.7
Brady, *Essentials of Paramedic Care*, 1st Edition, page 223.
Answer: D

112. Reference: DOT 5-2.8
Brady, *Essentials of Paramedic Care*, 1st Edition, pages 209 and 212.
Mosby, *Paramedic Textbook*, Revised 2nd Edition, page 757.
Answer: A

113. Reference: DOT 5-2.8
Brady, *Essentials of Paramedic Care*, 1st Edition, page 212.
Answer: A

114. Reference: DOT 5-2.7
Brady, *Essentials of Paramedic Care*, 1st Edition, page 1203.
Mosby, *Paramedic Textbook*, Revised 2nd Edition, page 756.
Answer: B

115. Reference: DOT 5-3.20
Brady, *Essentials of Paramedic Care*, 1st Edition, page 1369.
Answer: A

116. Reference: DOT 5-3.3
Brady, *Essentials of Paramedic Care*, 1st Edition, page 177.
Mosby, *Paramedic Textbook*, Revised 2nd Edition, pages 137-138.
Answer: C

117. Reference: DOT 5-3.3
Brady, *Essentials of Paramedic Care*, 1st Edition, page 177.
Mosby, *Paramedic Textbook*, Revised 2nd Edition, page 140.
Answer: B

118. Reference: DOT 5-3.3
Brady, *Essentials of Paramedic Care*, 1st Edition, pages 177-178.
Mosby, *Paramedic Textbook*, Revised 2nd Edition, page 911.
Answer: A

119. Reference: DOT 5-3.3
Brady, *Essentials of Paramedic Care*, 1st Edition, page 179.
Answer: D

120. Reference: DOT 5-3.3
Brady, *Essentials of Paramedic Care*, 1st Edition, page 179.
Mosby, *Paramedic Textbook*, Revised 2nd Edition, page 137.
Answer: C

121. Reference: DOT 5-4.1 and 5-4.36
Brady, *Essentials of Paramedic Care*, 1st Edition, page 1387.
Mosby, *Paramedic Textbook*, Revised 2nd Edition, pages 955-956.
Answer: B

122. Reference: DOT 5-4.3
Brady, *Essentials of Paramedic Care*, 1st Edition, page 1379.
Mosby, *Paramedic Textbook*, Revised 2nd Edition, page 945.
Answer: A

123. Reference: DOT 5-4.3
Brady, *Essentials of Paramedic Care*, 1st Edition, page 1379.
Answer: D

124. Reference: DOT 5-5.1
Brady, *Essentials of Paramedic Care*, 1st Edition, page 1395.
Mosby, *Paramedic Textbook*, Revised 2nd Edition, page 967.
Answer: A

125. Reference: DOT 5-5.2
Brady, *Essentials of Paramedic Care*, 1st Edition, page 1395.
Mosby, *Paramedic Textbook*, Revised 2nd Edition, page 1551.
Answer: A

126. Reference: DOT 5-6.1
Brady, *Essentials of Paramedic Care*, 1st Edition, page 1407.
Mosby, *Paramedic Textbook*, Revised 2nd Edition, page 977.
Answer: A

127. Reference: DOT 5-6.2
Brady, *Essentials of Paramedic Care*, 1st Edition, page 1412.
Answer: C

128. Reference: DOT 5-6.3
Brady, *Essentials of Paramedic Care*, 1st Edition, page 1419.
Answer: A

129. Reference: DOT 5-6.5
Brady, *Essentials of Paramedic Care*, 1st Edition, page 1408.
Answer: C

130. Reference: DOT 5-7.1
Brady, *Essentials of Paramedic Care*, 1st Edition, page 1432.
Mosby, *Paramedic Textbook*, Revised 2nd Edition, page 995.
Answer: D

131. Reference: DOT 5-7.2
Brady, *Essentials of Paramedic Care*, 1st Edition, page 249.
Answer: B

132. Reference: DOT 5-8.20 and 5-8.21
Brady, *Essentials of Paramedic Care*, 1st Edition, page 962.
Mosby, *Paramedic Textbook*, Revised 2nd Edition, page 610.
Answer: A

133. Reference: DOT 5-8.4
Brady, *Essentials of Paramedic Care*, 1st Edition, pages 1458 and 2013.
Mosby, *Paramedic Textbook*, Revised 2nd Edition, pages 1029-1030.
Answer: A

134. Reference: DOT 5-8
Mosby, *Paramedic Textbook*, Revised 2nd Edition, page 1001.
Answer: A

135. Reference: DOT 5-9.1
Brady, *Essentials of Paramedic Care*, 1st Edition, pages 120 and 122.
Answer: D

136. Reference: DOT 5-9.1
Brady, *Essentials of Paramedic Care*, 1st Edition, page 120.
Answer: A

137. Reference: DOT 5-10.1
Brady, *Essentials of Paramedic Care*, 1st Edition, page 1516.
Answer: A

138. Reference: DOT 5-10.2
Brady, *Essentials of Paramedic Care*, 1st Edition, page 1520.
Answer: D

139. Reference: DOT 5-10.3
Brady, *Essentials of Paramedic Care*, 1st Edition, page 1516.
Answer: C

140. Reference: DOT 5-10.4
Brady, *Essentials of Paramedic Care*, 1st Edition, page 1516.
Answer: C

141. Reference: DOT 5-11.1

Brady, *Essentials of Paramedic Care*, 1st Edition, pages 1503-1504 and 101.
Mosby, *Paramedic Textbook*, Revised 2nd Edition, page 153.
Answer: D

142. Reference: DOT 5-11.2

Brady, *Essentials of Paramedic Care*, 1st Edition, page 1557.
Mosby, *Paramedic Textbook*, Revised 2nd Edition, page 1108.
Answer: A

143. Reference: DOT 5-11.4

Brady, *Essentials of Paramedic Care*, 1st Edition, page 1557.
Mosby, *Paramedic Textbook*, Revised 2nd Edition, page 1102.
Answer: A

144. Reference: DOT 5-12.1

Brady, *Essentials of Paramedic Care*, 1st Edition, page 1607.
Answer: C

145. Reference: DOT 5-12.2

Brady, *Essentials of Paramedic Care*, 1st Edition, page 1607.
Mosby, *Paramedic Textbook*, Revised 2nd Edition, page 1145.
Answer: A

146. Reference: DOT 5-13.1

Brady, *Essentials of Paramedic Care*, 1st Edition, page 252.
Mosby, *Paramedic Textbook*, Revised 2nd Edition, page 992.
Answer: C

147. Reference: DOT 5-14.2

Brady, *Essentials of Paramedic Care*, 1st Edition, page 259.
Answer: D

148. Reference: DOT 6-2.35

Brady, *Essentials of Paramedic Care*, 1st Edition, page 833.
Mosby, *Paramedic Textbook*, Revised 2nd Edition, pages 535-536.
Answer: B

149. Reference: DOT 6-3.87

Brady, *Essentials of Paramedic Care*, 1st Edition, page 856.
Mosby, *Paramedic Textbook*, Revised 2nd Edition, page 1282 T43-1.
Answer: D

150. Reference: DOT 6-3.1

Brady, *Essentials of Paramedic Care*, 1st Edition, page 1800.
Mosby, *Paramedic Textbook*, Revised 2nd Edition, page 1278.
Answer: C

Don't forget to enter the information on your Personal Progress Plotter and answer the Yes and No question at the end of the Examination. This step is extremely important for the successful completion of the Systematic Approach to Examination Preparation!

Examination I-2 Answer Key

Directions
Follow these steps carefully for completing the feedback part of SAEP:

1. After calculating your score, look up the answers for the examination items you missed as well as those on which you guessed, even if you guessed correctly. If you are guessing, it means the answer is not perfectly clear. In this process, we are committed to making you as knowledgeable as possible.

2. Enter the number of missed and guessed examination items in the blanks on your Personal Progress Plotter.

3. Highlight the answer in the reference materials. Read the paragraph preceding and the paragraph following the one in which the correct answer is located. Enter the paragraph number and page number next to the guessed or missed examination item on your examination. Count any part of a paragraph at the beginning of the page as one paragraph until you reach the paragraph containing your highlighted answer. This step will help you locate and review your missed and guessed examination items later in the process. It is essential to learning the material in context and by association. These learning techniques (context/association) are the very backbone of the SAEP approach.

4. Once you have completed the feedback part, you may proceed to the next examination.

1. Reference: DOT 1-1.18
   Brady, *Essentials of Paramedic Care*, 1st Edition, page 8.
   Mosby, *Paramedic Textbook*, Revised 2nd Edition, page 22.
   Answer: B

2. Reference: DOT 1-1.21
   Brady, *Essentials of Paramedic Care*, 1st Edition, page 8.
   Answer: C

3. Reference: DOT 1-1.21
   Brady, *Essentials of Paramedic Care*, 1st Edition, page 8.
   Answer: B

4. Reference: DOT 1-1.22 and 1-1.33
   Brady, *Essentials of Paramedic Care*, 1st Edition, page 8.
   Answer: D

5. Reference: DOT 1-1.27
   Brady, *Essentials of Paramedic Care*, 1st Edition, page 8.
   Answer: D

6. Reference: DOT 1-2.21
   Brady, *Essentials of Paramedic Care*, 1st Edition, page 46.
   Answer: A

7. Reference: DOT 1-2.23
Brady, *Essentials of Paramedic Care*, 1st Edition, page 47.
Mosby, *Paramedic Textbook*, Revised 2nd Edition, page 44.
Answer: D

8. Reference: DOT 1-2.23
Brady, *Essentials of Paramedic Care*, 1st Edition, page 49.
Answer: A

9. Reference: DOT 1-3.9
Brady, *Essentials of Paramedic Care*, 1st Edition, page 58.
Mosby, *Paramedic Textbook*, Revised 2nd Edition, pages 60-61.
Answer: D

10. Reference: DOT 1-4.11
Brady, *Essentials of Paramedic Care*, 1st Edition, pages 79-81.
Mosby, *Paramedic Textbook*, Revised 2nd Edition, page 72.
Answer: B

11. Reference: DOT 1-4.27
Brady, *Essentials of Paramedic Care*, 1st Edition, page 92.
Mosby, *Paramedic Textbook*, Revised 2nd Edition, page 87.
Answer: D

12. Reference: DOT 1-4.13
Brady, *Essentials of Paramedic Care*, 1st Edition, page 82.
Mosby, *Paramedic Textbook*, Revised 2nd Edition, page 74.
Answer: D

13. Reference: DOT 1-4.14
Brady, *Essentials of Paramedic Care*, 1st Edition, page 82.
Answer: C

14. Reference: DOT 1-5.4
Brady, *Essentials of Paramedic Care*, 1st Edition, page 66.
Answer: B

15. Reference: DOT 1-6.11
Brady, *Essentials of Paramedic Care*, 1st Edition, page 287.
Mosby, *Paramedic Textbook*, Revised 2nd Edition, page 559.
Answer: C

16. Reference: DOT 1-6.12
Brady, *Essentials of Paramedic Care*, 1st Edition, page 293.
Mosby, *Paramedic Textbook*, Revised 2nd Edition, page 218.
Answer: D

17. Reference: DOT 1-6.12
Brady, *Essentials of Paramedic Care*, 1st Edition, page 294.
Mosby, *Paramedic Textbook*, Revised 2nd Edition, page 218.
Answer: A

18. Reference: DOT 1-6.12
Brady, *Essentials of Paramedic Care*, 1st Edition, page 293.
Mosby, *Paramedic Textbook*, Revised 2nd Edition, page 218.
Answer: A

19. Reference: DOT 1-6.13
Brady, *Essentials of Paramedic Care*, 1st Edition, page 298.
Mosby, *Paramedic Textbook*, Revised 2nd Edition, page 221.
Answer: B

20. Reference: DOT 1-7.25
Brady, *Essentials of Paramedic Care*, 1st Edition, page 410.
Mosby, *Paramedic Textbook*, Revised 2nd Edition, pages 1029-1030.
Answer: C

21. Reference: DOT 1-7.13
Brady, *Essentials of Paramedic Care*, 1st Edition, page 1244.
Mosby, *Paramedic Textbook*, Revised 2nd Edition, page 767.
Answer: C

22. Reference: DOT 1-7.13
Brady, *Essentials of Paramedic Care*, 1st Edition, page 217.
Mosby, *Paramedic Textbook*, Revised 2nd Edition, page 766.
Answer: C

23. Reference: DOT 1-7.13
Brady, *Essentials of Paramedic Care*, 1st Edition, pages 215-216.
Mosby, *Paramedic Textbook*, Revised 2nd Edition, page 761.
Answer: B

24. Reference: DOT 1-7.13
Brady, *Essentials of Paramedic Care*, 1st Edition, page 365.
Mosby, *Paramedic Textbook*, Revised 2nd Edition, page 932.
Answer: C

25. Reference: DOT 1-7.13
Brady, *Essentials of Paramedic Care*, 1st Edition, page 380.
Mosby, *Paramedic Textbook*, Revised 2nd Edition, page 1040.
Answer: C

26. Reference: DOT 1-8.24
Brady, *Essentials of Paramedic Care*, 1st Edition, page 416.
Mosby, *Paramedic Textbook*, Revised 2nd Edition, page 341.
Answer: B

27. Reference: DOT 1-8.8
Brady, *Essentials of Paramedic Care*, 1st Edition, page 473.
Mosby, *Paramedic Textbook*, Revised 2nd Edition, page 333.
Answer: B

28. Reference: DOT 1-8.8
Brady, *Essentials of Paramedic Care*, 1st Edition, page 474.
Mosby, *Paramedic Textbook*, Revised 2nd Edition, page 333.
Answer: D

29. Reference: DOT 1-8.8
Brady, *Essentials of Paramedic Care*, 1st Edition, page 475.
Answer: B

30. Reference: DOT 1-8.21
Brady, *Essentials of Paramedic Care*, 1st Edition, page 475.
Answer: C

31. Reference: DOT 1-8.9
Brady, *Essentials of Paramedic Care*, 1st Edition, page 480.
Mosby, *Paramedic Textbook*, Revised 2nd Edition, page 335.
Answer: A

32. Reference: DOT 1-9.5
Brady, *Essentials of Paramedic Care*, 1st Edition, page 582.
Mosby, *Paramedic Textbook*, Revised 2nd Edition, page 439.
Answer: A

33. Reference: DOT 1-9.9
Brady, *Essentials of Paramedic Care*, 1st Edition, page 583.
Answer: C

34. Reference: DOT 1-10.2
Brady, *Essentials of Paramedic Care*, 1st Edition, page 327.
Answer: C

35. Reference: DOT 1-10.3
Brady, *Essentials of Paramedic Care*, 1st Edition, page 327.
Answer: C

36. Reference: DOT 2-1.9
Brady, *Essentials of Paramedic Care*, 1st Edition, page 236.
Mosby, *Paramedic Textbook*, Revised 2nd Edition, pages 417 and 370.
Answer: A

37. Reference: DOT 2-1.14
Brady, *Essentials of Paramedic Care*, 1st Edition, page 231.
Answer: D

38. Reference: DOT 2-1.15
Brady, *Essentials of Paramedic Care*, 1st Edition, page 237.
Mosby, *Paramedic Textbook*, Revised 2nd Edition, page 389.
Answer: C

39. Reference: DOT 2-1.16
Brady, *Essentials of Paramedic Care*, 1st Edition, page 239.
Mosby, *Paramedic Textbook*, Revised 2nd Edition, page 201.
Answer: D

40. Reference: DOT 2-1.16
Brady, *Essentials of Paramedic Care*, 1st Edition, pages 239 and 267.
Answer: A

41. Reference: DOT 2-1.46
Brady, *Essentials of Paramedic Care*, 1st Edition, page 572.
Mosby, *Paramedic Textbook*, Revised 2nd Edition, pages 396-397.
Answer: B

42. Reference: DOT 2-1.47
Brady, *Essentials of Paramedic Care*, 1st Edition, page 566.
Mosby, *Paramedic Textbook*, Revised 2nd Edition, page 387.
Answer: B

43. Reference: DOT 2-1.73
Brady, *Essentials of Paramedic Care*, 1st Edition, page 528.
Answer: C

44. Reference: DOT 2-1.73
Brady, *Essentials of Paramedic Care*, 1st Edition, page 523.
Mosby, *Paramedic Textbook*, Revised 2nd Edition, page 408.
Answer: D

45. Reference: DOT 2-1.50
Brady, *Essentials of Paramedic Care*, 1st Edition, page 567.
Answer: C

46. Reference: DOT 3-1.3
Brady, *Essentials of Paramedic Care*, 1st Edition, page 592.
Mosby, *Paramedic Textbook*, Revised 2nd Edition, page 434.
Answer: B

47. Reference: DOT 3-2.23
Brady, *Essentials of Paramedic Care*, 1st Edition, page 647.
Mosby, *Paramedic Textbook*, Revised 2nd Edition, page 748.
Answer: A

48. Reference: DOT 3-2.24
Brady, *Essentials of Paramedic Care*, 1st Edition, page 617, Table 11-2.
Mosby, *Paramedic Textbook*, Revised 2nd Edition, page 385.
Answer: A

49. Reference: DOT 3-2.24
Brady, *Essentials of Paramedic Care*, 1st Edition, page 647.
Answer: D

50. Reference: DOT 3-2.59
Brady, *Essentials of Paramedic Care*, 1st Edition, page 695.
Mosby, *Paramedic Textbook*, Revised 2nd Edition, page 516.
Answer: B

51. Reference: DOT 3-2.59
Brady, *Essentials of Paramedic Care*, 1st Edition, page 696.
Mosby, *Paramedic Textbook*, Revised 2nd Edition, page 521.
Answer: C

52. Reference: DOT 3-2.60
Brady, *Essentials of Paramedic Care*, 1st Edition, page 1720.
Mosby, *Paramedic Textbook*, Revised 2nd Edition, pages 477-478.
Answer: B

53. Reference: DOT 3-3.28
Brady, *Essentials of Paramedic Care*, 1st Edition, pages 720-721.
Answer: D

54. Reference: DOT 3-3.29
Brady, *Essentials of Paramedic Care*, 1st Edition, page 721.
Mosby, *Paramedic Textbook*, Revised 2nd Edition, page 488.
Answer: D

55. Reference: DOT 3-3.30
Brady, *Essentials of Paramedic Care*, 1st Edition, page 694.
Mosby, *Paramedic Textbook*, Revised 2nd Edition, page 487.
Answer: B

56. Reference: DOT 3-3.41
Brady, *Essentials of Paramedic Care*, 1st Edition, page 744.
Mosby, *Paramedic Textbook*, Revised 2nd Edition, page 489.
Answer: C

57. Reference: DOT 3-3.37
Brady, *Essentials of Paramedic Care*, 1st Edition, page 744.
Answer: D

58. Reference: DOT 3-3.42
Brady, *Essentials of Paramedic Care*, 1st Edition, page 725.
Mosby, *Paramedic Textbook*, Revised 2nd Edition, page 715.
Answer: B

59. Reference: DOT 3-4.5
Brady, *Essentials of Paramedic Care*, 1st Edition, page 766.
Mosby, *Paramedic Textbook*, Revised 2nd Edition, pages 493-494.
Answer: A

60. Reference: DOT 3-4.7 and 3-4.3
Brady, *Essentials of Paramedic Care*, 1st Edition, page 767.
Mosby, *Paramedic Textbook*, Revised 2nd Edition, page 494.
Answer: D

61. Reference: DOT 3-5.16(e)
Brady, *Essentials of Paramedic Care*, 1st Edition, page 781.
Mosby, *Paramedic Textbook*, Revised 2nd Edition, page 508.
Answer: D

62. Reference: DOT 3-5.16(f)
Brady, *Essentials of Paramedic Care*, 1st Edition, page 781.
Answer: A

63. Reference: DOT 3-5.16(g)
Brady, *Essentials of Paramedic Care*, 1st Edition, page 782.
Answer: B

64. Reference: DOT 3-5.25
Brady, *Essentials of Paramedic Care*, 1st Edition, page 575.
Mosby, *Paramedic Textbook*, Revised 2nd Edition, page 502.
Answer: B

65. Reference: DOT 3-6.24
Brady, *Essentials of Paramedic Care*, 1st Edition, page 801.
Answer: D

66. Reference: DOT 3-6.23
Brady, *Essentials of Paramedic Care*, 1st Edition, page 801.
Answer: A

67. Reference: DOT 3-6.14
Brady, *Essentials of Paramedic Care*, 1st Edition, page 806.
Answer: D

68. Reference: DOT 3-6.14
Brady, *Essentials of Paramedic Care*, 1st Edition, page 807.
Answer: A

69. Reference: DOT 4-1
Brady, *Essentials of Paramedic Care*, 1st Edition, page 861.
Mosby, *Paramedic Textbook*, Revised 2nd Edition, page 546.
Answer: C

70. Reference: DOT 4-1
Brady, *Essentials of Paramedic Care*, 1st Edition, page 862.
Mosby, *Paramedic Textbook*, Revised 2nd Edition, page 545.
Answer: D

71. Reference: DOT 4-2.1
Brady, *Essentials of Paramedic Care*, 1st Edition, page 815.
Mosby, *Paramedic Textbook*, Revised 2nd Edition, page 527.
Answer: D

72. Reference: DOT 4-1.2
Brady, *Essentials of Paramedic Care*, 1st Edition, page 817.
Mosby, *Paramedic Textbook*, Revised 2nd Edition, page 529.
Answer: A

73. Reference: DOT 4-2.6 and 4-2.27
Brady, *Essentials of Paramedic Care*, 1st Edition, page 1730.
Mosby, *Paramedic Textbook*, Revised 2nd Edition, page 451.
Answer: D

74. Reference: DOT 4-2.7 and 4-2.44

Brady, *Essentials of Paramedic Care*, 1st Edition, page 902.
Mosby, *Paramedic Textbook*, Revised 2nd Edition, page 569.
Answer: C

75. Reference: DOT 4-2.8

Brady, *Essentials of Paramedic Care*, 1st Edition, page 449.
Answer: C

76. Reference: DOT 4-3.28 (A)

Brady, *Essentials of Paramedic Care*, 1st Edition, page 921.
Answer: C

77. Reference: DOT 4-3.11

Brady, *Essentials of Paramedic Care*, 1st Edition, page 915.
Mosby, *Paramedic Textbook*, Revised 2nd Edition, page 577.
Answer: D

78. Reference: DOT 4-3.27

Brady, *Essentials of Paramedic Care*, 1st Edition, page 857.
Answer: C

79. Reference: DOT 4-4.23, 4-4.20, and 4-4.29

Brady, *Essentials of Paramedic Care*, 1st Edition, pages 962 and 970.
Answer: B

80. Reference: DOT 4-4.22, 4-4.29, and 4-4.24

Brady, *Essentials of Paramedic Care*, 1st Edition, pages 964 and 971.
Mosby, *Paramedic Textbook*, Revised 2nd Edition, page 610.
Answer: D

81. Reference: DOT 4-4.40 and 4-4.41

Brady, *Essentials of Paramedic Care*, 1st Edition, page 979.
Mosby, *Paramedic Textbook*, Revised 2nd Edition, page 614.
Answer: B

82. Reference: DOT 4-4.45 and 4-4.41

Brady, *Essentials of Paramedic Care*, 1st Edition, page 957.
Answer: C

83. Reference: DOT 4-5.43

Brady, *Essentials of Paramedic Care*, 1st Edition, page 1037.
Answer: B

84. Reference: DOT 4-5.65

Brady, *Essentials of Paramedic Care*, 1st Edition, page 899.
Answer: A

85. Reference: DOT 4-5.46

Brady, *Essentials of Paramedic Care*, 1st Edition, page 1061.
Answer: B

86. Reference: DOT 4-5.46

Brady, *Essentials of Paramedic Care*, 1st Edition, page 1061.

Answer: C

87. Reference: DOT 4-6.4

Brady, *Essentials of Paramedic Care*, 1st Edition, page 1074.

Answer: D

88. Reference: DOT 4-6.3

Brady, *Essentials of Paramedic Care*, 1st Edition, page 1077.

Mosby, *Paramedic Textbook*, Revised 2nd Edition, pages 1406-1409.

Answer: C

89. Reference: DOT 4-6.19

Brady, *Essentials of Paramedic Care*, 1st Edition, page 1079.

Mosby, *Paramedic Textbook*, Revised 2nd Edition, page 489.

Answer: B

90. Reference: DOT 4-6.19

Brady, *Essentials of Paramedic Care*, 1st Edition, pages 185-186.

Mosby, *Paramedic Textbook*, Revised 2nd Edition, page 667.

Answer: B

91. Reference: DOT 8-2.36 and 1-1.31

Brady, *Essentials of Paramedic Care*, 1st Edition, page 1120.

Answer: A

92. Reference: DOT 4-7.6

Brady, *Essentials of Paramedic Care*, 1st Edition, page 1123.

Mosby, *Paramedic Textbook*, Revised 2nd Edition, page 458.

Answer: B

93. Reference: DOT 4-7.3

Brady, *Essentials of Paramedic Care*, 1st Edition, pages 1114-1115.

Mosby, *Paramedic Textbook*, Revised 2nd Edition, page 697.

Answer: D

94. Reference: DOT 4-7.23

Brady, *Essentials of Paramedic Care*, 1st Edition, page 1117.

Answer: D

95. Reference: DOT 4-8.2

Brady, *Essentials of Paramedic Care*, 1st Edition, page 242.

Answer: C

96. Reference: DOT 4-8.42

Brady, *Essentials of Paramedic Care*, 1st Edition, 1st Printing, page 1150.

Mosby, *Paramedic Textbook*, Revised 2nd Edition, page 566.

Answer: A

97. Reference: DOT 4-9.10
Brady, *Essentials of Paramedic Care*, 1st Edition, page 1005.
Mosby, *Paramedic Textbook*, Revised 2nd Edition, page 715.
Answer: B

98. Reference: DOT 4-9.12
Brady, *Essentials of Paramedic Care*, 1st Edition, page 1017.
Mosby, *Paramedic Textbook*, Revised 2nd Edition, page 718.
Answer: C

99. Reference: DOT 4-9.25
Brady, *Essentials of Paramedic Care*, 1st Edition, page 1017.
Mosby, *Paramedic Textbook*, Revised 2nd Edition, page 718.
Answer: C

100. Reference: DOT 4-9.25
Brady, *Essentials of Paramedic Care*, 1st Edition, page 1020.
Mosby, *Paramedic Textbook*, Revised 2nd Edition, page 1502.
Answer: C

101. Reference: DOT 5-1.5
Brady, *Essentials of Paramedic Care*, 1st Edition, page 1160.
Answer: A

102. Reference: DOT 5-1.5
Brady, *Essentials of Paramedic Care*, 1st Edition, page 1161.
Mosby, *Paramedic Textbook*, Revised 2nd Edition, page 1091.
Answer: D

103. Reference: DOT 5-1.9
Brady, *Essentials of Paramedic Care*, 1st Edition, page 1170.
Mosby, *Paramedic Textbook*, Revised 2nd Edition, page 417.
Answer: D

104. Reference: DOT 5-1.9
Brady, *Essentials of Paramedic Care*, 1st Edition, page 1171.
Answer: D

105. Reference: DOT 5-1.10(G)
Brady, *Essentials of Paramedic Care*, 1st Edition, page 1177.
Mosby, *Paramedic Textbook*, Revised 2nd Edition, page 746.
Answer: B

106. Reference: DOT 5-2.35 and 5-2.38
Brady, *Essentials of Paramedic Care*, 1st Edition, pages 1218 and 1225.
Mosby, *Paramedic Textbook*, Revised 2nd Edition, page 799.
Answer: C

107. Reference: DOT 5-2.35 and 5-2.38
Brady, *Essentials of Paramedic Care*, 1st Edition, page 1227.
Mosby, *Paramedic Textbook*, Revised 2nd Edition, pages 800-801.
Answer: C

108. Reference: DOT 5-2.37 and 5-2.50
Brady, *Essentials of Paramedic Care*, 1st Edition, pages 1221, 1239, and 1294.
Answer: C

109. Reference: DOT 5-2.39
Brady, *Essentials of Paramedic Care*, 1st Edition, page 1231.
Mosby, *Paramedic Textbook*, Revised 2nd Edition, pages 803-804.
Answer: D

110. Reference: DOT 5-2.35 and 5-2.39
Brady, *Essentials of Paramedic Care*, 1st Edition, page 1233.
Answer: D

111. Reference: DOT 5-2.52, 5-2.51, and 5-2.38
Brady, *Essentials of Paramedic Care*, 1st Edition, page 1221.
Mosby, *Paramedic Textbook*, Revised 2nd Edition, page 798.
Answer: A

112. Reference: DOT 5-2.51, 5-2.52, 5-2.53, and 5-2.162
Brady, *Essentials of Paramedic Care*, 1st Edition, page 1239.
Mosby, *Paramedic Textbook*, Revised 2nd Edition, pages 806-809.
Answer: B

113. Reference: DOT 5-2.50, 5-2.51, 5-2.52, and 5-2.162
Brady, *Essentials of Paramedic Care*, 1st Edition, page 1249.
Mosby, *Paramedic Textbook*, Revised 2nd Edition, page 850.
Answer: B

114. Reference: DOT 5-2.55, 5-2.54, and 5-2.162
Brady, *Essentials of Paramedic Care*, 1st Edition, page 1251.
Mosby, *Paramedic Textbook*, Revised 2nd Edition, page 855.
Answer: D

115. Reference: DOT 5-2.50, 5-2.53, and 5-2.52
Brady, *Essentials of Paramedic Care*, 1st Edition, page 1266.
Mosby, *Paramedic Textbook*, Revised 2nd Edition, page 829.
Answer: C

116. Reference: DOT 5-2.147
Brady, *Essentials of Paramedic Care*, 1st Edition, page 1336.
Answer: B

117. Reference: DOT 5-2.134
Brady, *Essentials of Paramedic Care*, 1st Edition, page 1207.
Mosby, *Paramedic Textbook*, Revised 2nd Edition, page 773.
Answer: D

118. Reference: DOT 5-2.34
Brady, *Essentials of Paramedic Care*, 1st Edition, page 1207.
Mosby, *Paramedic Textbook*, Revised 2nd Edition, page 773.
Answer: D

119. Reference: DOT 5-2.34

Brady, *Essentials of Paramedic Care*, 1st Edition, page 1337.
Mosby, *Paramedic Textbook*, Revised 2nd Edition, page 776.
Answer: B

120. Reference: DOT 5-2.20

Brady, *Essentials of Paramedic Care*, 1st Edition, pages 212-213.
Mosby, *Paramedic Textbook*, Revised 2nd Edition, pages 227-228.
Answer: D

121. Reference: DOT 5-3.18

Brady, *Essentials of Paramedic Care*, 1st Edition, page 1366.
Mosby, *Paramedic Textbook*, Revised 2nd Edition, page 1593.
Answer: C

122. Reference: DOT 5-3.20

Brady, *Essentials of Paramedic Care*, 1st Edition, pages 1366-1367.
Answer: B

123. Reference: DOT 5-3.22

Brady, *Essentials of Paramedic Care*, 1st Edition, page 1367.
Mosby, *Paramedic Textbook*, Revised 2nd Edition, page 934.
Answer: B

124. Reference: DOT 5-3.66(i)

Brady, *Essentials of Paramedic Care*, 1st Edition, page 1373.
Mosby, *Paramedic Textbook*, Revised 2nd Edition, page 939.
Answer: B

125. Reference: DOT 5-3.66(j)

Brady, *Essentials of Paramedic Care*, 1st Edition, page 1373.
Mosby, *Paramedic Textbook*, Revised 2nd Edition, page 940.
Answer: D

126. Reference: DOT 5-3.63

Brady, *Essentials of Paramedic Care*, 1st Edition, page 1373.
Mosby, *Paramedic Textbook*, Revised 2nd Edition, page 940.
Answer: A

127. Reference: DOT 5-4.26

Brady, *Essentials of Paramedic Care*, 1st Edition, page 1388.
Mosby, *Paramedic Textbook*, Revised 2nd Edition, pages 957-958.
Answer: C

128. Reference: DOT 5-4.24

Brady, *Essentials of Paramedic Care*, 1st Edition, page 1388.
Mosby, *Paramedic Textbook*, Revised 2nd Edition, page 955.
Answer: D

129. Reference: DOT 5-4.7

Brady, *Essentials of Paramedic Care*, 1st Edition, page 1393.
Answer: C

130. Reference: DOT 5-4.63
Brady, *Essentials of Paramedic Care*, 1st Edition, page 1392.
Answer: A

131. Reference: DOT 5-5.7
Brady, *Essentials of Paramedic Care*, 1st Edition, page 1399.
Mosby, *Paramedic Textbook*, Revised 2nd Edition, pages 225-226.
Answer: B

132. Reference: DOT 5-5.8
Brady, *Essentials of Paramedic Care*, 1st Edition, pages 1395 and 1399.
Answer: D

133. Reference: DOT 5-6-46
Brady, *Essentials of Paramedic Care*, 1st Edition, page 1425.
Answer: D

134. Reference: DOT 5-6.3
Brady, *Essentials of Paramedic Care*, 1st Edition, page 1425.
Answer: A

135. Reference: DOT 5-6.88 and 5-6.89
Brady, *Essentials of Paramedic Care*, 1st Edition, pages 1429 and 1422.
Answer: A

136. Reference: DOT 5-6.52
Brady, *Essentials of Paramedic Care*, 1st Edition, page 1419.
Answer: D

137. Reference: DOT 5-7.7
Brady, *Essentials of Paramedic Care*, 1st Edition, page 1439.
Mosby, *Paramedic Textbook*, Revised 2nd Edition, pages 994-995.
Answer: C

138. Reference: DOT 5-7.8
Brady, *Essentials of Paramedic Care*, 1st Edition, page 1441.
Answer: A

139. Reference: DOT 5-7.25
Brady, *Essentials of Paramedic Care*, 1st Edition, page 1452.
Answer: C

140. Reference: DOT 5-8.58
Brady, *Essentials of Paramedic Care*, 1st Edition, page 1484.
Mosby, *Paramedic Textbook*, Revised 2nd Edition, page 1023.
Answer: A

141. Reference: DOT 5-8.58
Brady, *Essentials of Paramedic Care*, 1st Edition, page 1403.
Mosby, *Paramedic Textbook*, Revised 2nd Edition, page 973.
Answer: C

142. Reference: DOT 5-8.58

Brady, *Essentials of Paramedic Care*, 1st Edition, page 1487.
Mosby, *Paramedic Textbook*, Revised 2nd Edition, page 1025.
Answer: A

143. Reference: DOT 5-9.15

Brady, *Essentials of Paramedic Care*, 1st Edition, page 127.
Mosby, *Paramedic Textbook*, Revised 2nd Edition, page 574.
Answer: B

144. Reference: DOT 5-9.22(b)

Brady, *Essentials of Paramedic Care*, 1st Edition, page 1510.
Answer: A

145. Reference: DOT 5-9.22(d)

Brady, *Essentials of Paramedic Care*, 1st Edition, pages 1499-1500.
Answer: A

146. Reference: DOT 4-4.47 and 4-4.54

Brady, *Essentials of Paramedic Care*, 1st Edition, page 1550.
Mosby, *Paramedic Textbook*, Revised 2nd Edition, page 619.
Answer: C

147. Reference: DOT 5-10.40 and 5-10.38

Brady, *Essentials of Paramedic Care*, 1st Edition, page 1529.
Mosby, *Paramedic Textbook*, Revised 2nd Edition, pages 1087-1088.
Answer: B

148. Reference: DOT 5-10.75

Brady, *Essentials of Paramedic Care*, 1st Edition, page 1546.
Answer: A

149. Reference: DOT 5-11.25

Brady, *Essentials of Paramedic Care*, 1st Edition, page 1579.
Answer: C

150. Reference: DOT 5-11.48

Brady, *Essentials of Paramedic Care*, 1st Edition, page 1597.
Mosby, *Paramedic Textbook*, Revised 2nd Edition, page 938.
Answer: C

Don't forget to enter the information on your Personal Progress Plotter and answer the Yes and No question at the end of the Examination. This step is extremely important for the successful completion of the Systematic Approach to Examination Preparation!

Examination I-3 Answer Key

Directions

Follow these steps carefully for completing the feedback part of SAEP:

1. After calculating your score, look up the answers for the examination items you missed as well as those on which you guessed, even if you guessed correctly. If you are guessing, it means the answer is not perfectly clear. In this process, we are committed to making you as knowledgeable as possible.

2. Enter the number of missed and guessed examination items in the blanks on your Personal Progress Plotter.

3. Highlight the answer in the reference materials. Read the paragraph preceding and the paragraph following the one in which the correct answer is located. Enter the paragraph number and page number next to the guessed or missed examination item on your examination. Count any part of a paragraph at the beginning of the page as one paragraph until you reach the paragraph containing your highlighted answer. This step will help you locate and review your missed and guessed examination items later in the process. It is essential to learning the material in context and by association. These learning techniques (context/association) are the very backbone of the SAEP approach.

4. Congratulations! You have completed the examination and feedback steps of SAEP when you have highlighted your guessed and missed examination items for this examination.

Proceed to Phases II and III. Study the materials carefully in these important phases—they will help you polish your examination-taking skills. Approximately two or three days before you take your next examination, carefully read all of the highlighted information in the reference materials using the same techniques you applied during the feedback step. This will reinforce your learning and provide you with an added level of confidence going into the examination.

Someone once said to professional golfer Tom Watson after he won several tournament championships, "You are really lucky to have won those championships. You are really on a streak." Watson was reported to have replied, "Yes, there is some luck involved, but what I have really noticed is that the more I practice, the luckier I get." What Watson was saying is that good luck usually results from good preparation. This line of thinking certainly applies to learning the rules and hints of examination taking.

—————— **Rule 7** ——————

Good luck = good preparation.

1. Reference: DOT 1-1.1(c)
   Brady, *Essentials of Paramedic Care*, 1st Edition, page 17.
   Mosby, *Paramedic Textbook*, Revised 2nd Edition, page 15.
   Answer: A

2. Reference: DOT 1-1.14
   Brady, *Essentials of Paramedic Care*, 1st Edition, page 12.
   Mosby, *Paramedic Textbook*, Revised 2nd Edition, page 6.
   Answer: B

3. Reference: DOT 1-1.32
Brady, *Essentials of Paramedic Care*, 1st Edition, page 21.
Mosby, *Paramedic Textbook*, Revised 2nd Edition, page 529.
Answer: A

4. Reference: DOT 1-2.8
Brady, *Essentials of Paramedic Care*, 1st Edition, page 35.
Mosby, *Paramedic Textbook*, Revised 2nd Edition, page 37, Box 2-4.
Answer: D

5. Reference: DOT 1-2.20
Brady, *Essentials of Paramedic Care*, 1st Edition, page 46.
Mosby, *Paramedic Textbook*, Revised 2nd Edition, page 42, Figure 2-2.
Answer: D

6. Reference: DOT 1-3.1
Brady, *Essentials of Paramedic Care*, 1st Edition, page 52.
Mosby, *Paramedic Textbook*, Revised 2nd Edition, page 527.
Answer: A

7. Reference: DOT 1-3.1
Brady, *Essentials of Paramedic Care*, 1st Edition, page 56.
Answer: D

8. Reference: DOT 1-3.9
Brady, *Essentials of Paramedic Care*, 1st Edition, page 58.
Mosby, *Paramedic Textbook*, Revised 2nd Edition, pages 60-61.
Answer: D

9. Reference: DOT 1-4.7(b)
Brady, *Essentials of Paramedic Care*, 1st Edition, page 90.
Mosby, *Paramedic Textbook*, Revised 2nd Edition, page 82.
Answer: D

10. Reference: DOT 1-4.7(c)
Brady, *Essentials of Paramedic Care*, 1st Edition, page 88.
Mosby, *Paramedic Textbook*, Revised 2nd Edition, page 78.
Answer: D

11. Reference: DOT 1-4.13
Brady, *Essentials of Paramedic Care*, 1st Edition, page 82.
Mosby, *Paramedic Textbook*, Revised 2nd Edition, page 74.
Answer: D

12. Reference: DOT 1-4.15
Brady, *Essentials of Paramedic Care*, 1st Edition, page 83.
Mosby, *Paramedic Textbook*, Revised 2nd Edition, page 75.
Answer: B

13. Reference: DOT 1-4.20
Brady, *Essentials of Paramedic Care*, 1st Edition, page 88.
Mosby, *Paramedic Textbook*, Revised 2nd Edition, page 78.
Answer: B

14. Reference: DOT 1-4.24
Brady, *Essentials of Paramedic Care*, 1st Edition, page 89.
Mosby, *Paramedic Textbook*, Revised 2nd Edition, page 1160.
Answer: D

15. Reference: DOT 1-4.7(b)
Brady, *Essentials of Paramedic Care*, 1st Edition, page 91.
Mosby, *Paramedic Textbook*, Revised 2nd Edition, page 82.
Answer: C

16. Reference: DOT 1-4.26
Brady, *Essentials of Paramedic Care*, 1st Edition, page 92.
Mosby, *Paramedic Textbook*, Revised 2nd Edition, page 85.
Answer: C

17. Reference: DOT 1-6.13
Brady, *Essentials of Paramedic Care*, 1st Edition, pages 298-299.
Mosby, *Paramedic Textbook*, Revised 2nd Edition, page 221.
Answer: A

18. Reference: DOT 1-6.14
Brady, *Essentials of Paramedic Care*, 1st Edition, pages 298-299.
Answer: B

19. Reference: DOT 1-6.15
Brady, *Essentials of Paramedic Care*, 1st Edition, page 323.
Answer: D

20. Reference: DOT 1-6.18
Brady, *Essentials of Paramedic Care*, 1st Edition, page 306.
Mosby, *Paramedic Textbook*, Revised 2nd Edition, page 222.
Answer: D

21. Reference: DOT 1-7.2
Brady, *Essentials of Paramedic Care*, 1st Edition, page 341.
Mosby, *Paramedic Textbook*, Revised 2nd Edition, page 234.
Answer: B

22. Reference: DOT 1-7.11
Brady, *Essentials of Paramedic Care*, 1st Edition, pages 346-347.
Mosby, *Paramedic Textbook*, Revised 2nd Edition, page 260.
Answer: C

23. Reference: DOT 1-7.12
Brady, *Essentials of Paramedic Care*, 1st Edition, pages 347-348.
Mosby, *Paramedic Textbook*, Revised 2nd Edition, page 314.
Answer: D

24. Reference: DOT 1-7.13
Brady, *Essentials of Paramedic Care*, 1st Edition, page 377
Mosby, *Paramedic Textbook*, Revised 2nd Edition, page 274.
Answer: C

25. Reference: DOT 1-7.13
Mosby, *Paramedic Textbook*, Revised 2nd Edition, page 764.
Answer: D

26. Reference: DOT 1-7.13
Brady, *Essentials of Paramedic Care*, 1st Edition, page 388.
Answer: D

27. Reference: DOT 1-7.13
Brady, *Essentials of Paramedic Care*, 1st Edition, page 399.
Answer: C

28. Reference: DOT 1-7.23
Brady, *Essentials of Paramedic Care*, 1st Edition, page 382.
Mosby, *Paramedic Textbook*, Revised 2nd Edition, page 278.
Answer: A

29. Reference: DOT 1-7.24 and 1-7.18
Brady, *Essentials of Paramedic Care*, 1st Edition, page 379.
Answer: D

30. Reference: DOT 1-7
Brady, *Essentials of Paramedic Care*, 1st Edition, page 1324.
Mosby, *Paramedic Textbook*, Revised 2nd Edition, page 892.
Answer: C

31. Reference: DOT 1-7.24
Brady, *Essentials of Paramedic Care*, 1st Edition, pages 1266-1267.
Mosby, *Paramedic Textbook*, Revised 2nd Edition, page 829.
Answer: A

32. Reference: DOT 1-8.5
Brady, *Essentials of Paramedic Care*, 1st Edition, pages 494-495.
Mosby, *Paramedic Textbook*, Revised 2nd Edition, page 312.
Answer: C

33. Reference: DOT 1-8.8
Brady, *Essentials of Paramedic Care*, 1st Edition, page 448.
Mosby, *Paramedic Textbook*, Revised 2nd Edition, page 324.
Answer: A

34. Reference: DOT 1-8.3
Brady, *Essentials of Paramedic Care*, 1st Edition, page 454.
Mosby, *Paramedic Textbook*, Revised 2nd Edition, page 312.
Answer: C

35. Reference: DOT 1-8.8 and 1-8.21
Brady, *Essentials of Paramedic Care*, 1st Edition, page 464.
Mosby, *Paramedic Textbook*, Revised 2nd Edition, page 329.
Answer: A

36. Reference: DOT 1-8.9
Brady, *Essentials of Paramedic Care*, 1st Edition, page 486.
Mosby, *Paramedic Textbook*, Revised 2nd Edition, page 335.
Answer: D

37. Reference: DOT 1-8.14
Brady, *Essentials of Paramedic Care*, 1st Edition, page 415.
Mosby, *Paramedic Textbook*, Revised 2nd Edition, page 315.
Answer: B

38. Reference: DOT 1-8.16
Brady, *Essentials of Paramedic Care*, 1st Edition, page 426.
Mosby, *Paramedic Textbook*, Revised 2nd Edition, pages 381-382.
Answer: C

39. Reference: DOT 1-8.17
Brady, *Essentials of Paramedic Care*, 1st Edition, pages 424-425.
Answer: C

40. Reference: DOT 1-8.19
Brady, *Essentials of Paramedic Care*, 1st Edition, pages 430-431.
Answer: D

41. Reference: DOT 1-8.21
Brady, *Essentials of Paramedic Care*, 1st Edition, pages 444-447.
Mosby, *Paramedic Textbook*, Revised 2nd Edition, page 322.
Answer: C

42. Reference: DOT 1-8.23
Brady, *Essentials of Paramedic Care*, 1st Edition, page 477.
Answer: B

43. Reference: DOT 1-9.1
Brady, *Essentials of Paramedic Care*, 1st Edition, page 575.
Mosby, *Paramedic Textbook*, Revised 2nd Edition, page 345.
Answer: C

44. Reference: DOT 1-9.5
Brady, *Essentials of Paramedic Care*, 1st Edition, page 583.
Mosby, *Paramedic Textbook*, Revised 2nd Edition, page 350.
Answer: B

45. Reference: DOT 1-9.7
Brady, *Essentials of Paramedic Care*, 1st Edition, page 582.
Mosby, *Paramedic Textbook*, Revised 2nd Edition, page 350.
Answer: C

46. Reference: DOT 2-1.3
Brady, *Essentials of Paramedic Care*, 1st Edition, page 227.
Mosby, *Paramedic Textbook*, Revised 2nd Edition, page 156.
Answer: A

47. Reference: DOT 2-1.17

Brady, *Essentials of Paramedic Care*, 1st Edition, page 239.
Mosby, *Paramedic Textbook*, Revised 2nd Edition, pages 376-377.
Answer: A

48. Reference: DOT 2-1.11

Brady, *Essentials of Paramedic Care*, 1st Edition, page 508.
Answer: A

49. Reference: DOT 2-1.4

Brady, *Essentials of Paramedic Care*, 1st Edition, page 231.
Mosby, *Paramedic Textbook*, Revised 2nd Edition, pages 159-160.
Answer: B

50. Reference: DOT 2-1.75

Brady, *Essentials of Paramedic Care*, 1st Edition, page 546.
Answer: C

51. Reference: DOT 2-1.4

Brady, *Essentials of Paramedic Care*, 1st Edition, page 235.
Answer: C

52. Reference: DOT 2-1.9

Brady, *Essentials of Paramedic Care*, 1st Edition, page 236.
Mosby, *Paramedic Textbook*, Revised 2nd Edition, pages 417 and 370.
Answer: A

53. Reference: DOT 2-1.19

Brady, *Essentials of Paramedic Care*, 1st Edition, page 239.
Answer: B

54. Reference: DOT 2-1.28

Brady, *Essentials of Paramedic Care*, 1st Edition, page 510.
Mosby, *Paramedic Textbook*, Revised 2nd Edition, page 408.
Answer: D

55. Reference: DOT 2-1.51

Brady, *Essentials of Paramedic Care*, 1st Edition, page 567.
Mosby, *Paramedic Textbook*, Revised 2nd Edition, page 388.
Answer: D

56. Reference: DOT 2-1.62

Brady, *Essentials of Paramedic Care*, 1st Edition, pages 510-511.
Mosby, *Paramedic Textbook*, Revised 2nd Edition, page 394.
Answer: B

57. Reference: DOT 2-1.65

Brady, *Essentials of Paramedic Care*, 1st Edition, pages 539-540.
Mosby, *Paramedic Textbook*, Revised 2nd Edition, page 422.
Answer: B

58. Reference: DOT 2-1.72
Brady, *Essentials of Paramedic Care*, 1st Edition, page 555.
Answer: A

59. Reference: DOT 3-1.2
Brady, *Essentials of Paramedic Care*, 1st Edition, page 580.
Mosby, *Paramedic Textbook*, Revised 2nd Edition, page 434.
Answer: D

60. Reference: DOT 3-1.5
Brady, *Essentials of Paramedic Care*, 1st Edition, page 594.
Mosby, *Paramedic Textbook*, Revised 2nd Edition, page 434.
Answer: C

61. Reference: DOT 3-2.14
Brady, *Essentials of Paramedic Care*, 1st Edition, page 637.
Answer: A

62. Reference: DOT 3-2.18
Brady, *Essentials of Paramedic Care*, 1st Edition, page 642.
Answer: C

63. Reference: DOT 3-2.24
Brady, *Essentials of Paramedic Care*, 1st Edition, page 617, Table 11-2.
Mosby, *Paramedic Textbook*, Revised 2nd Edition, page 385.
Answer: A

64. Reference: DOT 3-2.24
Brady, *Essentials of Paramedic Care*, 1st Edition, page 647.
Answer: D

65. Reference: DOT 3-2.25
Brady, *Essentials of Paramedic Care*, 1st Edition, page 648.
Answer: A

66. Reference: DOT 3-2.26
Brady, *Essentials of Paramedic Care*, 1st Edition, page 613.
Answer: B

67. Reference: DOT 3-2.29
Brady, *Essentials of Paramedic Care*, 1st Edition, page 652.
Answer: B

68. Reference: DOT 3-2.40
Brady, *Essentials of Paramedic Care*, 1st Edition, page 655.
Answer: A

69. Reference: DOT 3-2.4
Brady, *Essentials of Paramedic Care*, 1st Edition, page 815.
Mosby, *Paramedic Textbook*, Revised 2nd Edition, page 529.
Answer: B

70. Reference: DOT 3-3.12

Brady, *Essentials of Paramedic Care*, 1st Edition, page 1686.
Mosby, *Paramedic Textbook*, Revised 2nd Edition, page 1217.
Answer: A

71. Reference: DOT 3-3.39

Brady, *Essentials of Paramedic Care*, 1st Edition, page 727.
Mosby, *Paramedic Textbook*, Revised 2nd Edition, page 692.
Answer: B

72. Reference: DOT 3-3.12

Brady, *Essentials of Paramedic Care*, 1st Edition, page 714.
Answer: D

73. Reference: DOT 3-3.41

Brady, *Essentials of Paramedic Care*, 1st Edition, page 744.
Mosby, *Paramedic Textbook*, Revised 2nd Edition, page 489.
Answer: C

74. Reference: DOT 3-2.4

Brady, *Essentials of Paramedic Care*, 1st Edition, pages 777-778.
Mosby, *Paramedic Textbook*, Revised 2nd Edition, pages 433-434.
Answer: D

75. Reference: DOT 3-4.7 and 3-4.4

Brady, *Essentials of Paramedic Care*, 1st Edition, page 767.
Mosby, *Paramedic Textbook*, Revised 2nd Edition, pages 496-497.
Answer: D

76. Reference: DOT 3-4.7

Brady, *Essentials of Paramedic Care*, 1st Edition, page 767.
Mosby, *Paramedic Textbook*, Revised 2nd Edition, page 496.
Answer: C

77. Reference: DOT 3-5.15 and 3-5.17

Brady, *Essentials of Paramedic Care*, 1st Edition, page 775.
Mosby, *Paramedic Textbook*, Revised 2nd Edition, page 501.
Answer: B

78. Reference: DOT 3-5.13

Brady, *Essentials of Paramedic Care*, 1st Edition, page 782.
Answer: D

79. Reference: DOT 3-5.16(g)

Brady, *Essentials of Paramedic Care*, 1st Edition, page 782.
Answer: B

80. Reference: DOT 3-5.19, 3-5.21, and 3-5.20

Brady, *Essentials of Paramedic Care*, 1st Edition, page 776.
Answer: D

81. Reference: DOT 3-6.14
Brady, *Essentials of Paramedic Care*, 1st Edition, pages 803-804.
Answer: B

82. Reference: DOT 3-6.23
Brady, *Essentials of Paramedic Care*, 1st Edition, page 801.
Answer: A

83. Reference: DOT 4-1.12
Brady, *Essentials of Paramedic Care*, 1st Edition, pages 829-830.
Answer: A

84. Reference: DOT 4-1.7
Brady, *Essentials of Paramedic Care*, 1st Edition, page 847.
Mosby, *Paramedic Textbook*, Revised 2nd Edition, page 540.
Answer: B

85. Reference: DOT 4-1
Brady, *Essentials of Paramedic Care*, 1st Edition, page 864.
Answer: A

86. Reference: DOT 4-1.3
Brady, *Essentials of Paramedic Care*, 1st Edition, page 822.
Answer: A

87. Reference: DOT 5-1.3
Brady, *Essentials of Paramedic Care*, 1st Edition, page 234.
Mosby *Paramedic Textbook*, Revised 2nd Edition, page 363.
Answer: A

88. Reference: DOT 4-2.16
Brady, *Essentials of Paramedic Care*, 1st Edition, page 879.
Answer: D

89. Reference: DOT 4-2.2
Brady, *Essentials of Paramedic Care*, 1st Edition, page 880.
Mosby, *Paramedic Textbook*, Revised 2nd Edition, page 574.
Answer: A

90. Reference: DOT 4-2.43
Brady, *Essentials of Paramedic Care*, 1st Edition, page 288.
Mosby, *Paramedic Textbook*, Revised 2nd Edition, page 564.
Answer: A

91. Reference: DOT 4-2.8
Brady, *Essentials of Paramedic Care*, 1st Edition, page 904.
Mosby, *Paramedic Textbook*, Revised 2nd Edition, page 569.
Answer: C

92. Reference: DOT 4-3.4
Brady, *Essentials of Paramedic Care*, 1st Edition, pages 916-917.
Answer: A

93. Reference: DOT 4-3.12 (D)
Brady, *Essentials of Paramedic Care*, 1st Edition, page 918.
Mosby, *Paramedic Textbook*, Revised 2nd Edition, page 580.
Answer: A

94. Reference: DOT 4-3.24
Brady, *Essentials of Paramedic Care*, 1st Edition, page 928.
Mosby, *Paramedic Textbook*, Revised 2nd Edition, page 583.
Answer: D

95. Reference: DOT 4-3.26
Brady, *Essentials of Paramedic Care*, 1st Edition, pages 915 and 928.
Answer: B

96. Reference: DOT 4-3.38
Brady, *Essentials of Paramedic Care*, 1st Edition, page 926.
Answer: A

97. Reference: DOT 4-3.40
Brady, *Essentials of Paramedic Care*, 1st Edition, page 923.
Mosby, *Paramedic Textbook*, Revised 2nd Edition, page 593.
Answer: B

98. Reference: DOT 4-3.42
Brady, *Essentials of Paramedic Care*, 1st Edition, page 828.
Answer: A

99. Reference: DOT 4-3-18 and 4-3.20
Brady, *Essentials of Paramedic Care*, 1st Edition, page 849.
Answer: D

100. Reference: DOT 4-4.7 and 4-4.5
Brady, *Essentials of Paramedic Care*, 1st Edition, page 974.
Mosby, *Paramedic Textbook*, Revised 2nd Edition, page 602.
Answer: D

101. Reference: DOT 4-4.3
Brady, *Essentials of Paramedic Care*, 1st Edition, page 955.
Answer: A

102. Reference: DOT 4-4.3
Brady, *Essentials of Paramedic Care*, 1st Edition, page 955.
Mosby, *Paramedic Textbook*, Revised 2nd Edition, pages 598-599.
Answer: C

103. Reference: DOT 4-4.7 and 4-4.5
Brady, *Essentials of Paramedic Care*, 1st Edition, pages 973-974.
Answer: B

104. Reference: DOT 4-4.40 and 4-4.41
Brady, *Essentials of Paramedic Care*, 1st Edition, page 979.
Mosby, *Paramedic Textbook*, Revised 2nd Edition, page 614.
Answer: B

105. Reference: DOT 4-5.34
Brady, *Essentials of Paramedic Care*, 1st Edition, page 1067.
Answer: B

106. Reference: DOT 4-5.36
Brady, *Essentials of Paramedic Care*, 1st Edition, pages 179-181.
Answer: D

107. Reference: DOT 4-5.39 and 4-5.52
Brady, *Essentials of Paramedic Care*, 1st Edition, page 1030.
Answer: C

108. Reference: DOT 4-5.65
Brady, *Essentials of Paramedic Care*, 1st Edition, page 899.
Answer: A

109. Reference: DOT 4-5.46
Brady, *Essentials of Paramedic Care*, 1st Edition, page 1058.
Answer: D

110. Reference: DOT 4-6
Brady, *Essentials of Paramedic Care*, 1st Edition, page 185.
Answer: A

111. Reference: DOT 4-6.14
Brady, *Essentials of Paramedic Care*, 1st Edition, page 1082.
Answer: B

112. Reference: DOT 4-6.35
Brady, *Essentials of Paramedic Care*, 1st Edition, page 1088.
Mosby, *Paramedic Textbook*, Revised 2nd Edition, pages 678-679.
Answer: B

113. Reference: DOT 4-6.19
Brady, *Essentials of Paramedic Care*, 1st Edition, pages 185-186.
Mosby, *Paramedic Textbook*, Revised 2nd Edition, page 667.
Answer: B

114. Reference: DOT 4-6.15
Brady, *Essentials of Paramedic Care*, 1st Edition, page 1078.
Mosby, *Paramedic Textbook*, Revised 2nd Edition, page 668.
Answer: B

115. Reference: DOT 4-7.21 and 4-7.21(A)
Brady, *Essentials of Paramedic Care*, 1st Edition, pages 838-839.
Answer: A

116. Reference: DOT 4-6.2
Brady, *Essentials of Paramedic Care*, 1st Edition, page 238.
Mosby, *Paramedic Textbook*, Revised 2nd Edition, page 375.
Answer: A

117. Reference: DOT 4-3.14 and 4-3.12(J)

Brady, *Essentials of Paramedic Care*, 1st Edition, page 865.
Mosby, *Paramedic Textbook*, Revised 2nd Edition, pages 543 and 1102.
Answer: C

118. Reference: DOT 4-7.9(B)

Brady, *Essentials of Paramedic Care*, 1st Edition, page 1107.
Mosby, *Paramedic Textbook*, Revised 2nd Edition, page 688.
Answer: A

119. Reference: DOT 4-7.14

Brady, *Essentials of Paramedic Care*, 1st Edition, page 1112
Mosby, *Paramedic Textbook*, Revised 2nd Edition, page 695.
Answer: D

120. Reference: DOT 4-7.17(A)

Brady, *Essentials of Paramedic Care*, 1st Edition, page 1115.
Mosby, *Paramedic Textbook*, Revised 2nd Edition, page 697.
Answer: A

121. Reference: DOT 4-7.18

Brady, *Essentials of Paramedic Care*, 1st Edition, page 1114.
Answer: B

122. Reference: DOT 4-8.2

Brady, *Essentials of Paramedic Care*, 1st Edition, page 245.
Answer: C

123. Reference: DOT 4-8.2

Brady, *Essentials of Paramedic Care*, 1st Edition, page 246.
Mosby, *Paramedic Textbook*, Revised 2nd Edition, page 290.
Answer: C

124. Reference: DOT 4-8.2

Brady, *Essentials of Paramedic Care*, 1st Edition, page 1138.
Mosby, *Paramedic Textbook*, Revised 2nd Edition, pages 704-706.
Answer: C

125. Reference: DOT 4-9.2

Brady, *Essentials of Paramedic Care*, 1st Edition, page 130.
Mosby, *Paramedic Textbook*, Revised 2nd Edition, page 125.
Answer: A

126. Reference: DOT 4-9.2

Brady, *Essentials of Paramedic Care*, 1st Edition, page 131.
Answer: B

127. Reference: DOT 4-9.10

Brady, *Essentials of Paramedic Care*, 1st Edition, page 1005.
Mosby, *Paramedic Textbook*, Revised 2nd Edition, page 715.
Answer: B

128. Reference: DOT 5-1.3
Brady, *Essentials of Paramedic Care*, 1st Edition, page 239.
Mosby, *Paramedic Textbook*, Revised 2nd Edition, page 367.
Answer: A

129. Reference: DOT 5-1.3
Brady, *Essentials of Paramedic Care*, 1st Edition, page 238.
Mosby, *Paramedic Textbook*, Revised 2nd Edition, pages 375-376.
Answer: A

130. Reference: DOT 5-1.5
Brady, *Essentials of Paramedic Care*, 1st Edition, page 1167.
Mosby, *Paramedic Textbook*, Revised 2nd Edition, page 458.
Answer: D

131. Reference: DOT 5-1.9
Brady, *Essentials of Paramedic Care*, 1st Edition, page 1170.
Mosby, *Paramedic Textbook*, Revised 2nd Edition, page 417.
Answer: D

132. Reference: DOT 5-1.10(B)
Brady, *Essentials of Paramedic Care*, 1st Edition, page 1182.
Answer: C

133. Reference: DOT 5-1.5
Brady, *Essentials of Paramedic Care*, 1st Edition, page 1189.
Answer: A

134. Reference: DOT 5-2.8
Brady, *Essentials of Paramedic Care*, 1st Edition, page 212.
Answer: A

135. Reference: DOT 5-2.11 and 5-2.12
Brady, *Essentials of Paramedic Care*, 1st Edition, page 218.
Mosby, *Paramedic Textbook*, Revised 2nd Edition, page 767.
Answer: A

136. Reference: DOT 5-2.32
Brady, *Essentials of Paramedic Care*, 1st Edition, page 1216.
Mosby, *Paramedic Textbook*, Revised 2nd Edition, pages 782-783.
Answer: D

137. Reference: DOT 5-2.31
Brady, *Essentials of Paramedic Care*, 1st Edition, pages 1209-1210.
Mosby, *Paramedic Textbook*, Revised 2nd Edition, page 781.
Answer: D

138. Reference: DOT 5-2.37
Brady, *Essentials of Paramedic Care*, 1st Edition, pages 1219-1220.
Mosby, *Paramedic Textbook*, Revised 2nd Edition, page 794.
Answer: A

139. Reference: DOT 5-2.38

Brady, *Essentials of Paramedic Care*, 1st Edition, page 1218.
Answer: D

140. Reference: DOT 5-2.35 and 5-2.38

Brady, *Essentials of Paramedic Care*, 1st Edition, page 1227.
Mosby, *Paramedic Textbook*, Revised 2nd Edition, pages 800-801.
Answer: C

141. Reference: DOT 5-2.35 and 5-2.39

Brady, *Essentials of Paramedic Care*, 1st Edition, page 1241.
Mosby, *Paramedic Textbook*, Revised 2nd Edition, pages 812-813.
Answer: B

142. Reference: DOT 5-2.39

Brady, *Essentials of Paramedic Care*, 1st Edition, page 1259.
Mosby, *Paramedic Textbook*, Revised 2nd Edition, page 807.
Answer: C

143. Reference: DOT 5-2.38

Brady, *Essentials of Paramedic Care*, 1st Edition, page 1263.
Mosby, *Paramedic Textbook*, Revised 2nd Edition, page 822.
Answer: D

144. Reference: DOT 5-2.35

Brady, *Essentials of Paramedic Care*, 1st Edition, pages 1264-1265.
Mosby, *Paramedic Textbook*, Revised 2nd Edition, pages 823-828.
Answer: C

145. Reference: DOT 5-2.75

Brady, *Essentials of Paramedic Care*, 1st Edition, pages 1313-1314.
Answer: D

146. Reference: DOT 5-2.77 and 5-2.76

Brady, *Essentials of Paramedic Care*, 1st Edition, page 1311.
Mosby, *Paramedic Textbook*, Revised 2nd Edition, pages 869-871.
Answer: A

147. Reference: DOT 5-2.94 and 5-2.95

Brady, *Essentials of Paramedic Care*, 1st Edition, page 1326.
Answer: B

148. Reference: DOT 5-2.100

Brady, *Essentials of Paramedic Care*, 1st Edition, page 1320.
Answer: C

149. Reference: DOT 5-2.114

Brady, *Essentials of Paramedic Care*, 1st Edition, page 1324.
Mosby, *Paramedic Textbook*, Revised 2nd Edition, pages 882-883.
Answer: C

150. Reference: DOT 5-2.115
Brady, *Essentials of Paramedic Care*, 1st Edition, page 1325.
Answer: C

151. Reference: DOT 5-2.133
Brady, *Essentials of Paramedic Care*, 1st Edition, page 1331.
Mosby, *Paramedic Textbook*, Revised 2nd Edition, pages 81-82.
Answer: C

152. Reference: DOT 5-2.142
Mosby, *Paramedic Textbook*, Revised 2nd Edition, pages 886-887.
Answer: B

153. Reference: DOT 5-3.3
Brady, *Essentials of Paramedic Care*, 1st Edition, page 169.
Mosby, *Paramedic Textbook*, Revised 2nd Edition, page 139.
Answer: D

154. Reference: DOT 5-3.3
Brady, *Essentials of Paramedic Care*, 1st Edition, page 182.
Mosby, *Paramedic Textbook*, Revised 2nd Edition, page 133.
Answer: C

155. Reference: DOT 5-3.10
Brady, *Essentials of Paramedic Care*, 1st Edition, page 1364.
Mosby, *Paramedic Textbook*, Revised 2nd Edition, page 933.
Answer: B

156. Reference: DOT 5-3.20
Brady, *Essentials of Paramedic Care*, 1st Edition, pages 1366-1367.
Answer: B

157. Reference: DOT 5-3.25
Brady, *Essentials of Paramedic Care*, 1st Edition, page 1370.
Answer: D

158. Reference: DOT 5-3.25
Brady, *Essentials of Paramedic Care*, 1st Edition, page 1369.
Answer: C

159. Reference: DOT 5-3.51
Brady, *Essentials of Paramedic Care*, 1st Edition, page 1356.
Mosby, *Paramedic Textbook*, Revised 2nd Edition, page 929.
Answer: B

160. Reference: DOT 5-3.66(a)
Brady, *Essentials of Paramedic Care*, 1st Edition, page 1371.
Mosby, *Paramedic Textbook*, Revised 2nd Edition, page 936.
Answer: B

161. Reference: DOT 5-4.3
Brady, *Essentials of Paramedic Care*, 1st Edition, page 198.
Mosby, *Paramedic Textbook*, Revised 2nd Edition, page 145.
Answer: D

162. Reference: DOT 5-4.19 and 5-4.30
Brady, *Essentials of Paramedic Care*, 1st Edition, page 1385.
Answer: B

163. Reference: DOT 5-4.43
Brady, *Essentials of Paramedic Care*, 1st Edition, page 1385.
Mosby, *Paramedic Textbook*, Revised 2nd Edition, page 956.
Answer: D

164. Reference: DOT 5-4.32
Brady, *Essentials of Paramedic Care*, 1st Edition, page 1386.
Mosby, *Paramedic Textbook*, Revised 2nd Edition, page 958.
Answer: A

165. Reference: DOT 5-4.46
Brady, *Essentials of Paramedic Care*, 1st Edition, pages 1385-1387.
Mosby, *Paramedic Textbook*, Revised 2nd Edition, page 956.
Answer: D

166. Reference: DOT 5-4.37
Brady, *Essentials of Paramedic Care*, 1st Edition, page 1384.
Mosby, *Paramedic Textbook*, Revised 2nd Edition, pages 956-957.
Answer: C

167. Reference: DOT 5-4.56
Brady, *Essentials of Paramedic Care*, 1st Edition, page 1391.
Answer: D

168. Reference: DOT 5-4.6
Brady, *Essentials of Paramedic Care*, 1st Edition, page 1391.
Answer: C

169. Reference: DOT 5-4.7
Brady, *Essentials of Paramedic Care*, 1st Edition, page 1393.
Answer: C

170. Reference: DOT 5-5.15
Brady, *Essentials of Paramedic Care*, 1st Edition, page 1400.
Mosby, *Paramedic Textbook*, Revised 2nd Edition, page 971.
Answer: D

171. Reference: DOT 5-6-43
Brady, *Essentials of Paramedic Care*, 1st Edition, page 1422.
Answer: D

172. Reference: DOT 5-6.50
   Brady, *Essentials of Paramedic Care*, 1st Edition, page 1417.
   Mosby, *Paramedic Textbook*, Revised 2nd Edition, page 984.
   Answer: D

173. Reference: DOT 5-6.62
   Brady, *Essentials of Paramedic Care*, 1st Edition, page 1421.
   Mosby, *Paramedic Textbook*, Revised 2nd Edition, page 985.
   Answer: C

174. Reference: DOT 5-7.16
   Brady, *Essentials of Paramedic Care*, 1st Edition, page 1446.
   Answer: D

175. Reference: DOT 5-8.21
   Brady, *Essentials of Paramedic Care*, 1st Edition, page 1457.
   Mosby, *Paramedic Textbook*, Revised 2nd Edition, page 1016, Table 34-1.
   Answer: C

176. Reference: DOT 5-8.10
   Brady, *Essentials of Paramedic Care*, 1st Edition, pages 1459-1460.
   Answer: D

177. Reference: DOT 5-8.12
   Brady, *Essentials of Paramedic Care*, 1st Edition, page 1457.
   Mosby, *Paramedic Textbook*, Revised 2nd Edition, page 1003.
   Answer: A

178. Reference: DOT 5-8.18
   Brady, *Essentials of Paramedic Care*, 1st Edition, page 1462.
   Mosby, *Paramedic Textbook*, Revised 2nd Edition, page 1004.
   Answer: D

179. Reference: DOT 5-8.58
   Brady, *Essentials of Paramedic Care*, 1st Edition, page 1482.
   Mosby, *Paramedic Textbook*, Revised 2nd Edition, page 1022.
   Answer: D

180. Reference: DOT 5-8.55
   Brady, *Essentials of Paramedic Care*, 1st Edition, page 1495.
   Mosby, *Paramedic Textbook*, Revised 2nd Edition, page 1050.
   Answer: C

181. Reference: DOT 5-9.7
   Brady, *Essentials of Paramedic Care*, 1st Edition, page 1506.
   Mosby, *Paramedic Textbook*, Revised 2nd Edition, page 1066.
   Answer: A

182. Reference: DOT 5-9.22(d)
   Brady, *Essentials of Paramedic Care*, 1st Edition, page 1508.
   Answer: D

183. Reference: DOT 5-10.4

Brady, *Essentials of Paramedic Care*, 1st Edition, page 1516.
Answer: C

184. Reference: DOT 5-10.44

Brady, *Essentials of Paramedic Care*, 1st Edition, page 1533.
Mosby, *Paramedic Textbook*, Revised 2nd Edition, pages 1088-1089.
Answer: A

185. Reference: DOT 5-10.57

Brady, *Essentials of Paramedic Care*, 1st Edition, pages 1535 and 1537.
Answer: B

186. Reference: DOT 5-10.67

Brady, *Essentials of Paramedic Care*, 1st Edition, page 1541.
Answer: C

187. Reference: DOT 5-10.78

Brady, *Essentials of Paramedic Care*, 1st Edition, pages 1546-1547.
Mosby, *Paramedic Textbook*, Revised 2nd Edition, page 1097.
Answer: D

188. Reference: DOT 5-11.2

Brady, *Essentials of Paramedic Care*, 1st Edition, page 1557.
Mosby, *Paramedic Textbook*, Revised 2nd Edition, page 1108.
Answer: A

189. Reference: DOT 5-11.24

Brady, *Essentials of Paramedic Care*, 1st Edition, page 1578.
Answer: A

190. Reference: DOT 5-11.27

Brady, *Essentials of Paramedic Care*, 1st Edition, page 1584.
Mosby, *Paramedic Textbook*, Revised 2nd Edition, pages 1123-1124.
Answer: C

191. Reference: DOT 5-11.29

Brady, *Essentials of Paramedic Care*, 1st Edition, page 1596.
Answer: D

192. Reference: DOT 5-11.39

Brady, *Essentials of Paramedic Care*, 1st Edition, page 1590.
Mosby, *Paramedic Textbook*, Revised 2nd Edition, pages 1132-1133.
Answer: C

193. Reference: DOT 5-11.48

Brady, *Essentials of Paramedic Care*, 1st Edition, page 1597.
Mosby, *Paramedic Textbook*, Revised 2nd Edition, page 938.
Answer: C

194. Reference: DOT 5-12.8(E)
Brady, *Essentials of Paramedic Care*, 1st Edition, page 1617.
Mosby, *Paramedic Textbook*, Revised 2nd Edition, page 1145.
Answer: B

195. Reference: DOT 5-12.19
Brady, *Essentials of Paramedic Care*, 1st Edition, page 1619.
Mosby, *Paramedic Textbook*, Revised 2nd Edition, page 1157.
Answer: A

196. Reference: DOT 5-13.4
Brady, *Essentials of Paramedic Care*, 1st Edition, page 1637.
Answer: D

197. Reference: DOT 5-13.3
Brady, *Essentials of Paramedic Care*, 1st Edition, page 1631.
Answer: B

198. Reference: DOT 5-14.13
Brady, *Essentials of Paramedic Care*, 1st Edition, page 1667.
Mosby, *Paramedic Textbook*, Revised 2nd Edition, page 1200.
Answer: C

199. Reference: DOT 5-14.16
Brady, *Essentials of Paramedic Care*, 1st Edition, pages 1667-1668.
Mosby, *Paramedic Textbook*, Revised 2nd Edition, pages 1200-1201.
Answer: A

200. Reference: DOT 6-2.35
Brady, *Essentials of Paramedic Care*, 1st Edition, page 833.
Mosby, *Paramedic Textbook*, Revised 2nd Edition, pages 535-536.
Answer: B

Don't forget to enter the information on your Personal Progress Plotter and answer the Yes and No question at the end of the Examination. This step is extremely important for the successful completion of the Systematic Approach to Examination Preparation!

Bibliography for Exam Prep: Paramedic

1. DOT National Standard Curriculum for EMT-Paramedic, 1998

2. Brady, *Essentials of Paramedic Care*, 1st Edition, 2002

3. Mosby, *Paramedic Textbook*, Revised 2nd Edition, 2001